The Yoga Adventure
for Children

SmartFun Books from Hunter House

101 Music Games for Children by Jerry Storms

101 More Music Games for Children by Jerry Storms

101 Dance Games for Children by Paul Rooyackers

101 More Dance Games for Children by Paul Rooyackers

101 Movement Games for Children by Huberta Wiertsema

101 Drama Games for Children by Paul Rooyackers

101 More Drama Games for Children by Paul Rooyackers

101 Improv Games for Children by Bob Bedore

101 Language Games for Children by Paul Rooyackers

101 Life Skills Games for Children by Bernie Badegruber

101 More Life Skills Games for Children by Bernie Badegruber

101 Cool Pool Games for Children by Kim Rodomista

101 Family Vacation Games by Shando Varda

404 Deskside Activities for Energetic Kids by Barbara Davis

Yoga Games for Children by Danielle Bersma and Marjoke Visscher

The Yoga Adventure for Children by Helen Purperhart

Ordering

Trade bookstores in the U.S. and Canada please contact:

Publishers Group West
1700 Fourth Street, Berkeley CA 94710
Phone: (800) 788-3123   Fax: (510) 528-3444

Hunter House books are available at bulk discounts for textbook course adoptions; to qualifying community, health-care, and government organizations; and for special promotions and fund-raising. For details please contact:

Special Sales Department
Hunter House Inc., PO Box 2914, Alameda CA 94501-0914
Phone: (510) 865-5282   Fax: (510) 865-4295
E-mail: ordering@hunterhouse.com

Individuals can order our books from most bookstores, by calling
(800) 266-5592, or from our Web site at **www.hunterhouse.com**

The
Yoga Adventure

Children

Playing, Dancing, Moving,
Breathing, Relaxing

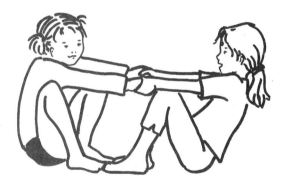

Helen Purperhart

Translated by Amina Marix Evans
Illustrated by Barbara van Amelsfort

A Hunter House Smart*Fun* Book

Hunter House Inc., Publishers
PO Box 2914
Alameda, CA 94501-0914

Library of Congress Cataloging-in-Publication Data

Purperhart, Helen.
[Het yoga avontuur voor kinderen. English]
The yoga adventure for children : playing, dancing, moving,
breathing, relaxing / Helen Purperhart.
p. cm. — (Yoga games for children)
ISBN-13: 978-0-89793-470-1 (pbk.)
ISBN-10: 0-89793-470-9 (pbk.)
ISBN-13: 978-0-89793-471-8 (spiral bound)
ISBN-10: 0-89793-471-7 (spiral bound)
1. Hatha yoga for children. I. Title.
RA781.7.P88 2006
613.7'046083—dc22   2006020292

Project Credits

Cover Design: Jil Weil and Stefanie Gold   Senior Marketing Associate: Reina Santana
Illustration: Barbara van Amelsfort   Rights Coordinator: Candace Groskreutz
Book Production: Stefanie Gold   Customer Service Manager:
Translator: Amina Marix Evans   Christina Sverdrup
Developmental & Copy Editor: Christy Steele   Order Fulfillment: Washul Lakdhon
Proofreader: Herman Leung   Administrator: Theresa Nelson
Acquisitions Editor: Jeanne Brondino   Computer Support: Peter Eichelberger
Editor: Alexandra Mummery   Publisher: Kiran S. Rana

Printed and Bound by Bang Printing, Brainerd, Minnesota

Manufactured in the United States of America

9 8 7 6 5 4 3 2 1   First Edition   07 08 09 10 11

Contents

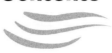

*A detailed list of the games indicating appropriate age
groups begins on the next page.*

List of Games

Important Note

The material in this book is intended to provide information about a safe, enjoyable exercise program for children. Every effort has been made to provide accurate and dependable information. The contents of this book have been compiled through professional research and in consultation with professionals. However, professionals have differing opinions, and some of the information may become outdated; therefore, the publisher, authors, and editors, as well as the professionals quoted in the book cannot be held responsible for any error, omission, or dated material. The authors and publisher assume no responsibility for any outcome of applying the information in this book. Follow the instructions closely. Note that children's bodies are fragile, so they should not be forced to assume any physical positions that cause them pain or discomfort. If you have questions concerning your exercise program or about the application of the information described in this book, consult a qualified professional.

Foreword

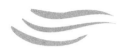

Helen came into the African dance class with shining eyes and a broad smile. From the moment the drums began, she was unstoppable. It was wonderful to watch her dancing; she moved like a forest goddess and offered her own contribution to the class.

When Helen told me she was pregnant, I felt enormously drawn to the new little being inside her. Carmel was born the day before my own birthday—two Cancers found each other. From that moment on, Helen and I decided to join forces. Our passion for dance, her yoga and games, and my own creativity turned out to be a unique combination. Helen and I taught each other a lot. We showed each other alternative ways of doing things. It has been wonderful to openly and honestly teach each other. From me, Helen has learned to keep certain things for herself, and she has taught me how to more efficiently deal with things.

Three years ago, we founded BuitelendePurperTraining. We used this name for our dance, drama, and drawing training because of the combination of our surnames and the symbolism of our combined efforts. During our first dance workshop, we were tested. Everything was progressing fine—good music and events happening just as we had agreed. The only thing we had not discussed was cleaning up afterward. It happened automatically, without us noticing it. The following evening, I discovered that the cash box was missing. A disappointed feeling came over us. Fortunately our feelings did not turn into blame, and equally fortunately, I found the box safely stowed under the driver's seat of the car. It became a good metaphor—we should invest in our dreams and passions instead of sitting on our money.

Our workshops are also our lessons for life. During her children's yoga course, she included a day for me to show her students the rudiments of how one can be creative by drawing and modeling in clay. This is an important way to help the children find creative ways of dealing with their ideas and gain insight into their own methods of self-expression. Previously, people had been concerned only with the task at hand. They didn't realize how much information was hidden in the individual's creativity. Through discussing this aspect with children, a door opens into a whole new world of self-awareness. The children become able to answer their own questions about their process, perhaps through drawing. It is important to be able to make this creativity clear to children.

This book nicely supplements all the yoga books currently available. Children are introduced to yoga in a very readable way. Helen's passion for yoga shines through her writing, and she explains the exercises in her own natural way. She also makes it clear that everyone can be creative when putting their yoga classes together. Her method of working with children shows a deep respect for youngsters of every color. Her unbridled energy and power prevent her from stopping until she is truly content or has achieved her goal. She is a fast worker and good at organizing—in short, great to work with. We both feel that we have won one of life's lotteries by finding one another.

— Emeke Buitelaar
July 13, 2003

About the Author

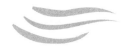

After completing my education in youth welfare work and social sciences in 1990, I went to work at a school for problem children in Amsterdam. While I was pregnant in 1992, I was inspired by yoga after being introduced to yoga for pregnancy. I continued with my study of yoga after my daughter was born. The idea of doing yoga for children formed when my daughter Nina, then five years old, wanted to do yoga classes. Since there were no yoga classes for children where we lived, I decided to create a children's yoga course myself. During this time, I learned how to combine yoga and playing. The games and drama projects that I had learned while studying welfare work were very useful.

When I saw the effect yoga had on children, I began the yoga center Jip & Jan in Almere, a town close to Amsterdam. Nina thought up the name for herself. She confused yin and yang with the children's book characters Jip and Janneke (pronounced Yip and Yanneke). When she saw the yin-yang sign, she cried, "Look, Mama, Yip and Yan!" And I thought it was a nice name for the future yoga center. Through my younger daughter, Carmel, I discovered that yoga is also suitable for young children. She is also crazy about yoga and spontaneously takes up the dog posture and starts singing when the mantra of compassion, *Om mani padme hum,* is played.

I also give yoga lessons at the school for problem children in Amsterdam, where I still work. A constant stream of disturbing thoughts plagues the youngsters who attend this school. They think about the distressing things that have happened to them, extremely tiring things they cannot let go of in their minds. The most important purpose of the yoga lesson is to help them become aware of these invasions. It is only when they see what is happening in their heads that they can begin to master their thoughts. During the lessons, I place a strong emphasis on discussing their experiences so that they gain more insight into their own situation. Yoga can be very therapeutic, but that is not the motivation for my lessons. Enjoyment is by far the most important element.

I have been teaching the children's yoga course for almost five years. Many of the people who have followed the course tell me enthusiastically that they use elements of the children's yoga method during their classes with adults. I frequently hear them say, "It is very liberating and much more fun than adult yoga," and, "It brings out the child in me."

African dance is another passion of mine. You have already "met" Emeke Buitelaar in her Foreword. Together we instruct teachers of children's yoga and do the BuitelendePurperTraining for teachers and group leaders in schools and kindergartens. The BuitelendePurperTraining is a combination of dance, drama, and drawing training.

Acknowledgments

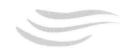

I dedicate this book to Marc Leeser and my daughters, Nina and Carmel. They continue to inspire and support me as I journey along the path to my goal.

I also dedicate it to my mother, Wil Purperhart, and my late father, Orlando Purperhart. They helped to make me who I am. Loving thanks to all who inspired me: Barbara van Amelsfort, who drew the illustrations with a great deal of humor and inspiration; Emeke Buitelaar, with whom I share wonderful adventures on the path to my self-development; Tanja Secreve, who introduced me to yoga during my pregnancy; and Ruurd Fenenga, who taught me the basics of Raja yoga. When I wanted to read my manuscript to Ruurd at the end of November last year, I heard that he had died peacefully on October 30, 2003. I often think about the enthusiastic and inspiring way he taught. I would also like to thank Bernadette Frets from the yoga institute Osmose, who helped me become familiar with the most important yoga postures and the different yoga techniques; Marjoke Visscher from Samsara Yoga Opleidingen, who showed me how to combine games with yoga; Ajata Stam from Levensschool Govindadhama, who helped me with the descriptions of the yoga rules for life; Sophie van der Zee, who helped translate the book into the child's world; Marion Gravendaal, Robert-Jan ter Beek, and Cynthia Stuger, who gave me positive feedback as I was working on the book.

Finally, I would like to thank all the children and adults who have taken part in my children's yoga courses. They continue to inspire and surprise me. It was a great adventure to be able to make this book, and it would never have come to fruition without the help of all these wonderful people.

Introduction

Children's yoga is not new. In fact, as information about its health and spiritual benefits continues to spread, it is attracting more and more interest. The aim of *The Yoga Adventure for Children* is to present a light-hearted way for both children and adults to familiarize themselves with yoga.

This book is written for yoga teachers, activity-group leaders, elementary-school teachers, and parents who are looking for fun ways to experience fitness with their children. Yoga promotes physical health and vitality, and many children who participate in yoga experience a healthy physical enjoyment. To encourage this, the book offers many creative games and exercises with suggestions for combining yoga with play. Children's yoga can be integrated between lessons in the classroom, during a gym class, or after school.

Spiritual exploration can be another aspect of yoga. Older children, in particular, enjoy self-reflection. Yoga can help them examine how their behavior can influence their lives. Yoga does not have answers for all the children's questions, however. Parents and teachers will need to help children find answers on their spiritual journey. Not all parents and teachers are spiritually oriented, so it should be noted that yoga can be taught without the spiritual element. Even without this element, yoga can be a useful tool for getting children to discuss things and to help them in their development.

The Exercises

The games in this book are organized into sections. Each section addresses a different aspect or principle of yoga. The games have been grouped into a section by their main focus. Some of the exercises, however, might be applicable for several sections. For example, a gentle yoga posture might also be used as a warming-up exercise.

Most of the exercises in this book are accompanied by drawings. These drawings will sometimes serve simply as illustrations, so be sure to follow the written instructions. Many of the exercises and stories are printed in italics and can be read verbatim to the children.

Planning the Yoga Class

Each of the yoga games can stand alone. However, you can also create a children's yoga class by selecting several games from the different sections of this book. A children's yoga lesson needs to be a dynamic affair with plenty of variety. Sitting still for long periods can cause boredom and irritation. By varying the activities during the class, the children remain absorbed and interested.

For instance, begin with a warming-up game to loosen the body. Then, offer a meditation exercise or a concentration exercise to help calm the children from the busyness of their day. Next, yoga postures will help make their bodies strong and supple. Consider adding a game for fun. Then encourage their imaginations with a story or a visualization exercise. Finally, a wake-up exercise will bring the children back to an alert state.

The instructions given in the book are only suggestions and are far from the only ways of playing the games. We invite you to be creative.

Timing

Yoga can be done anytime during the day; each time has its advantages. Yoga in the morning generates energy to begin the day. Yoga during school can refresh children and help them concentrate better on the lessons that follow. Doing yoga before going to bed can help children wind down and prepare for beautiful dreams. The children themselves, with the consent of their parents, can decide whether they want to do yoga in the morning, afternoon, or evening.

Yoga should not be done on a full stomach, so it should not be done right after lunch or right after dinner. It is recommended that you wait about 90 minutes after children have eaten a meal before having them do yoga.

A yoga class can be of varying lengths. Keep it enjoyable and be sensitive to the different abilities and physical limitations of each child. At school, setting aside an hour each week in the curriculum for yoga is sufficient. At home, the children can do the exercises for as long as they enjoy them, but as parents it is wise to make some limits—until supper or after they finish their homework, etc.

Workspace

Yoga doesn't require a special space. It can be done indoors or outside if the weather permits. For yoga in school, it is best to choose a space that is large enough so that everyone has enough room to move their arms about freely in all directions without touching another child. It is also best to find a room that is quiet and has minimal potential for distractions. An empty classroom, the gym, or recreation rooms are all potential yoga spaces. At home, the children can choose a place where they can be quiet and concentrate on their yoga.

Yoga is best performed with bare feet, which give children a good grip. At school, however, it may be preferable to wear shoes to avoid exposure to foot diseases and other germs. Children can use gym shoes or slippers with anti-slip soles. For floor exercises, a soft surface is better than a hard surface. Rubber mats can provide both warmth and good grip during yoga games, but they are optional.

Preparation

It is important to carefully prepare lessons. Before beginning, think about how to begin the class, where to stand, what to say (rules, agreements, duration of the games, signals to stop), and what might go wrong. Gather everything needed for the class in advance. Harmonize the lesson with the atmosphere the children bring with them. This may mean that the lesson takes a different path from the one you envisioned. For this reason, it is always a good idea to have a couple of extra exercises in reserve in case some do not work well.

You can choose whether or not to do the exercises with the children. Participation depends on the exercise, the group, and your goal. One advantage of participating is that it helps motivate the children. One disadvantage is that you are less able to monitor what the children are doing.

The Role of the Leader

Enjoyment should be the priority with children's yoga. To encourage this, the teacher should be enthusiastic and take a positive approach to the exercises. Focus on the things the children are doing right. This will pass on a positive attitude to them.

In order to facilitate this, keep analyzing why the children are behaving in a specific way. If there are children who don't want to participate in a certain exercise, don't try to force them. Children should be accepted as they are, even if they don't dare or don't want to do some things.

Some of the exercises provide opportunities for experimentation. Encourage the children to express themselves. Encourage creativity. Compliment the children who express original ideas. As teacher, you may discover possibilities you had never realized.

Rules

It is important to offer clarity and structure in each yoga lesson. Children prefer to know in advance what they will be doing in a yoga class. At school, provide clear rules about what is allowed or not allowed during the lesson. When giving yoga lessons outside the school, make agreements that serve as rules of the game. Before you start the classes, put these rules on paper and give them to the parents. This way, both the children and parents are aware of the rules before the children's yoga group begins.

The five most common rules are as follows:

1. No eating during the class. It is distracting and can also be dangerous with certain exercises.
2. No wearing jewelry. Jewelry may get lost or broken or could hurt someone else.
3. Use the bathroom before class begins. This way, you won't have to leave during the lesson. (If necessary, schedule a toilet break in the middle of the lesson.)
4. Wear loose clothing, if possible. If you only have regular school clothes, loosen your belt.
5. Never move farther into a position than is comfortable for you. Yoga should feel good, not bad.

Duration

The duration of the games and length of time a child holds the posture will vary. Remember that children are fragile. Don't have them hold a posture for too long because this may damage their growing bodies. Children can discover their own limits by focusing on whether an exercise still feels good. It is best to let them choose for themselves whether to continue holding a posture or to stop.

Key to the Icons Used in the Games

To help you find games suitable for a particular situation, the games are coded with symbols or icons. These icons tell you at a glance some things about the game:

- The appropriate age group
- The size of the group needed
- If props are required

- If a large space is needed
- If physical contact is or might be involved

These are explained in more detail below.

Suitability in terms of age. The games are designed for children ages 4 through 12. The recommended age groups correspond to grade level divisions commonly used in the educational system.

 = Young children in preschool through grade 2 (ages 4–8)

 = All children in preschool through grade 6 (ages 4–12)

 = Children in grade 1 through grade 6 (ages 6–12)

 = Children in grade 3 through grade 6 (ages 8–12)

The size of the group needed. While some games require partners, you can play many of the games with any sized group.

 = Players will work in pairs

 = Players will work in small groups of three or more

If large space is needed. Almost all yoga games may be played in a small space. However, a large space is ideal for some of the games. The few games that require a large amount of space are marked with the following icon:

 = Large space needed

If props are required. Many of the games require no special props. In some cases, though, items such as balloons, crystals, or other objects are integral to running and playing a game. Games requiring props are flagged with the following icon, and the necessary materials are listed under the Props heading.

 = Props needed

If music is required. Only a few games in this book require the playing of recorded music. Several games include suggestions for suitable music. For instance, we might recommend music with Eastern themes or African drums.

 = Music required

If physical contact is or might be involved. Although a certain amount of body contact might be acceptable in certain environments, the following icon has been inserted at the top of any exercises that might involve anywhere from a small amount of contact to minor collisions. You can figure out in advance if the game is suitable for your participants and/or environment.

 = Physical contact likely

The Rules of Yoga

Yoga is an ancient art that was already in existence for several thousand years before people began counting. The word yoga means "binding." Yoga helps people bind together the physical, mental, and spiritual elements of their lives. Over time, people began to view body and soul as more of a single unit. This point of view led to the development of meditation techniques and methods for living a healthier life. Yoga became a part of daily life for many people.

The unity of knowledge and technique can be termed yoga. The traditional scriptures of yoga contain the multitude of yoga sutras, or teachings. Patanjali, the father of yoga, wrote the best-known scriptures in the ancient Indian language Sanskrit. The scriptures consist of short texts that communicate the essence of yoga. They also offer advice about different issues, including abstinence and one's function in society and relationship with oneself.

Many children are more interested in the philosophy behind the rules of yoga, rather than in the rules themselves. Yoga philosophy is based on the concept that people are connected with every other living thing on Earth and even in the universe, including people, animals, plants, earth, air, or water. Those who neglect their bodies are neglecting a part of Mother Nature, and those who think only of themselves are neglecting their self-development.

The book *Yoga Education for Children* by Swami Satyananda Saraswati contains the following piece about growing through yoga. It is adapted slightly so that older children can understand it well. The passage provides a clear account of what yoga represents:

> When you want to plant a garden with flowers and trees, what do you do first? Do you just sprinkle seeds? Many people might do that, but not much would grow. First you have to prepare the ground. You break up the earth and pull out the weeds. Then you can plant the seeds, and they will grow into beautiful flowers and trees. The same goes for the human spirit. Just like the earth, the spirit needs to be prepared in order to allow things to grow.
>
> In life, you meet many types of people. The things you tell them don't always sink in because their spirits have not been prepared for planting. Their spirit is still like hard soil, so things cannot grow well, no matter how hard you work on it. There are also people whose spirits are like soft soil. When you tell these people something, their spirits

soak it up like sponges. Practicing yoga is like working on your own garden so that the quality of your consciousness is able to develop. If a person has a spirit with good soil and without weeds, all kinds of things may be planted and grown.

Without the philosophy, yoga would be very similar to gymnastics. Yet yoga is far more than that. It is a way of life. In the following sections, yoga philosophy is adapted to the experience of a child.

The Five Abstinences

One of the rules of yoga concerns abstinence. The rule is divided into five different abstinences. People should avoid all kinds of bad habits regarding violence, lying, theft, and desire. These are universal moral commandments concerning the outer world.

1. Nonviolence

The first abstinence is the development of a nonviolent attitude to life. People learn to recognize their own anger, aggression, and ignorance. By examining what makes them angry, people can distance themselves from it. By accepting themselves, people give themselves the space to change. They become more loving and more able to restrain themselves from causing pain to other people or things.

In this increasingly violent world, it becomes ever more important to encourage nonviolence in children. There are different ways to do this. People can reduce or completely eliminate the amount of violence and aggression children watch on television. The same, of course, applies to video games. Teaching children how to deal with anger, aggression, and bullying is another important task. Recent research shows that hitting a punching bag or a cushion, for instance, can help children express their anger without hurting anyone. Parents and teachers should listen to what children say about the cause of their anger—of course this is possible only after the child has calmed down a bit.

2. Truth and Honesty

The second abstinence is about speaking the truth and conducting one's life accordingly. Lying will not solve problems. People can encourage honesty in children by talking to them about lying and its consequences. Don't be too quick to punish children if they honestly tell about something you would rather not hear. Instead, praise them for their honesty, and tell them how much you appreciate it. Recognize how hard it is for them to tell you about it.

3. Not Stealing

The third abstinence is about not stealing. Children should learn not to take anything that does not belong to them. This doesn't just mean theft of objects, but also stealing other people's ideas. Encourage children to have their own ideas and compliment them for their originality. Honesty creates more trust from other people, and honesty with oneself creates more self-confidence.

4. Self-Control

The fourth abstinence is about greed and sensuality. It is an important type of abstinence, particularly for pubescent children. During this phase of life, hormonal changes make their sexual desires much stronger, so it is very important to practice self-control. The same applies to enjoyment of food and drink, especially alcohol. Here, too, children can teach themselves not to take more than they need.

5. Nonpossessiveness

The fifth abstinence is about distancing oneself from greed. For many children, the amount of possessions their friends have is very important, and they usually don't want to have fewer things themselves. This often means more toys, expensive clothes, a faster computer, or video games. Talk with children about their personal needs in terms of clothes, food, and even attention. Teach them the difference between wanting something and truly needing something.

The Five Precepts

Another part of yoga philosophy is formed by the five precepts. The precepts are five habits for healthy self-development. People develop and improve themselves through practicing purity, contentment, self-discipline, self-directed learning, and devotion.

1. Purity

The first precept is about cleanliness of the body, food, and surroundings. It is also about cleanliness in thoughts, words, and actions. Adults can be good examples by living a clean life, eating healthy foods, caring for the environment, and not speaking negatively about other people in front of children.

2. Contentment

The second precept is about being content with what you have. Striving for improvement is still acceptable, but people realize that improvement comes from dedication to humanity, animals, plants, earth, air, and water. People become happier by improving themselves and by being kind, not by accumulating more possessions. By avoiding moaning in front of the children about the need for a bigger house, more free time, etc., adults can serve as an example.

3. Austerity (Self-discipline)

Austerity is the third precept, which helps children develop positive habits. A child could, for instance, pledge to practice yoga for a certain length of time at a particular hour each day. Perhaps a child could decide to eat fewer sweets. Adults can help children identify some aspect of their lives where they can practice self-discipline. The emphasis should be on helping them. Don't tell them exactly what they should do when it comes to self-discipline, and once they have made a decision regarding a habit, don't constantly remind them about what they have decided to do because doing so might create a negative focus.

4. Self-Directed Learning

Self-directed learning is the fourth precept. It is about instructing the self, not just by doing homework or reading books. Children who regularly ponder such questions as "Who am I?" and "What is my purpose?" will find it easier to apply the rules of yoga in their own lives. Adults can guide children in finding answers by giving them books to read or encouraging them to keep a journal of their thoughts. Of course, it is important that the children also want to do it.

5. Devotion

Devotion is the fifth, and most important, precept. It is about dedication to the spiritual life, which is not driven by individual wishes and desires. Adults can make this subject easier to talk about by emphasizing how children should be confident in their own strength and believe that they are fine just as they are.

The Peace Agreement

The Buddhist monk Thich Nhat Hanh devised a peace agreement to encourage nonviolence. The peace agreement is a practical development of the first abstinence of nonviolence.

The agreement on the next page has been adapted for use with children. By carefully reading it, children will acquire a different view of anger. Before they look for a solution to a conflict, you can advise children to examine whether they have been unkind and made the other person sad or angry. Or ask them if they have short-changed themselves. Make as many photocopies of the agreement as needed to use for conflicts at school or at home.

THE PEACE AGREEMENT

_____

and

_____

declare that if we have disagreements, we will work on finding a solution to the problem by using the following rules and conditions:

- We will say and do nothing to make the disagreement worse.
- We will let the other person know within a day, and quietly, that you are angry.
- We will work together to find a solution to the problem in the short term.
- We will postpone agreements about solving the problem if the anger remains.
- We will have respect for each other's feelings, and give each other enough time to calm down.
- We will listen to each other, and don't interrupt.
- We won't bring other issues into the argument. Keep to the point.
- We will not judge the other person and will take their explanation seriously.
- We will offer our apologies as soon as we understand what went wrong.
- We won't try to absolve ourselves of blame.

_____   _____

NAME   NAME

_____   _____

DATE   DATE

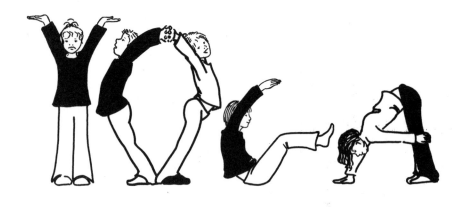

Exercises, Games, and Stories

Warm-Up Exercises—
Dance of the Joints

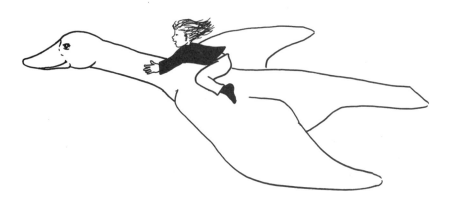

This section contains short warm-up exercises to prepare the mind and body for yoga. Warming up will help muscles get ready for physical activity and reduce the risk of injury.

These warm-up exercises have several important benefits. First, they will increase the body's muscle temperature, making them supple and pliable for yoga. Participants' heart rate and respiratory rate will slowly increase. As a result, blood flow to the muscles and joints increases. The increased flow of oxygen and nutrients to muscles helps prepare them for more strenuous yoga activity.

The games in Dance of the Joints will increase flexibility and help make children more aware of the role each joint has in their bodies. Many of the games require children to stand up or balance on one leg. Children who find this difficult can hold on to a chair or lean against the wall for support.

The games are best accompanied by music with Eastern themes. The movements will flow into one another in time to the music, creating a dance.

Fingers

Instruct the children as follows: *Stand up and face forward. Hold your left hand in front of your chest with the palm facing upward. With your right hand, take hold of the little finger of your left hand. Breathe in deeply. As you breathe in, bend the little finger gently backward. Next, exhale. As you exhale, let the finger slowly move upward into its original position.*

Have the children repeat these moves on each finger of the left hand. Then have them repeat the moves on the fingers of the right hand.

Note: This game is best accompanied by music with Eastern themes.

Wrists

Tell the children: *Stand up and face forward. Hold your hands in front of your heart. Make circles with your wrists, first one way and then the other. Do this ten times in each direction.*

When you are done, shake your wrists and hands until they feel nice and loose.

Note: This game is best accompanied by music with Eastern themes.

3

Knees

Guide the children as follows: *Stand up and face forward. Slowly bend your right leg. Then, reach down and hold your right thigh with your hands. Lift your right foot off the ground until your knee is pointing straight ahead. Rotate your lower leg at*

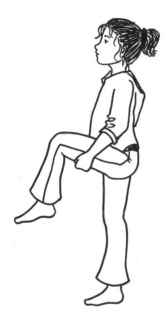

the knee ten times to the left. Next, rotate your lower leg at the knee ten times to the right. Repeat the exercise with your left leg.

Note: This game is best accompanied by music with Eastern themes.

Feet

Say to the children: *Stand up and face forward. Bend your right leg. Reach down and hold your lower right leg with your hands. Now lift your right foot from the ground. Turn it in circles to the left ten times. Then, turn it in circles to the right ten times. Repeat these movements with the left foot.*

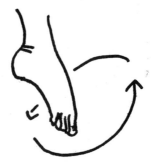

Note: This game is best accompanied by music with Eastern themes.

5

Hips

Instruct the children as follows: *Stand up straight with your hands by your sides. Make clockwise circles with your hips. To do this, first move your hips forward; then to the right; next backward; finally, finish the circle by moving your hips to the left.*

Now do ten counterclockwise circles with your hips. To do this, first move your hips backward; then to the left; next forward; finally, finish the circle by moving your hips to the right.

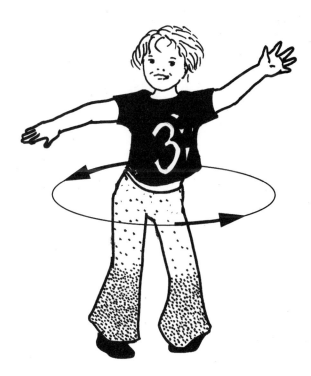

Notes

- Demonstrate the exercise before asking the children to do it. This will ensure that the children are moving their hips in the correct direction.
- This game is best accompanied by music with Eastern themes.

Yoga Postures

Yoga postures are both fun and useful. Yoga can help children either to recharge their energy or to burn off excess energy.

Children should be able to steadily and comfortably hold each posture. Practicing the postures helps make their bodies strong and supple. Postures relax their bodies and make their muscles firm.

Sun Salutation

The sun salutation, explained on the next two pages, is a series of yoga postures performed in a sequence with inhalations and exhalations. The postures are arranged so that every part of the body is exercised. Each posture stretches or flexes the spine so that the entire body becomes supple and elastic. The movements flow into each other, stimulating energy and enhancing circulation.

This series is an effective warm-up, or each posture of the sun salutation can also stand alone as a separate exercise.

6

Sun Salutation

Read each instruction aloud:

- *Stand up straight with your feet together. Bring your palms together in front of your chest with your fingers pointing upward.*

- *Breathe in and stretch your arms above your head. Bend your head backward slightly and look upward.*

- *Breathing out, bend forward. Keep your legs straight, and touch the ground with your fingertips. Bring your face as close to your knees as you can. If you can't touch the ground with your knees straight, then bend them slightly.*

- *Breathing in, look straight in front. Step back with your right foot. Your toes should touch the ground and point forward.*

- *Breathing out, step back with your left foot. Push your heels as far as possible to the ground. Look at your navel.*

- *Breathing in, bend your arms and slowly sink to the floor. Touch the floor with your hands, chest, knees, and toes. Look downward.*

- *As you breathe in, stretch and stiffen your arms. Use them to lift the upper part of your body from the floor. Gently bend your spine backward in an arch. Bend your head back and look upward.*

- *Put your toes firmly on the ground. As you exhale, raise the middle of your body and push your bottom in the air. Keeping your hands and feet on the ground, look at your navel.*

- *Breathing in, bend your right leg forward. Keep your left leg stretched out behind you and look forward.*

- *Breathing out, step forward with your left leg. Straighten both legs. Touch your fingertips to the ground. Hold your face as closely as possible to your knees.*

- *As you breathe in, slowly straighten your spine and raise yourself to a standing position again, leading the movement with your arms straight out. Stretch your arms upward. Bend your head backward a little and look upward.*

- *As you breathe out, bring your hands together in front of your chest. Close your eyes. Continue breathing in and out softly and slowly open your eyes.*

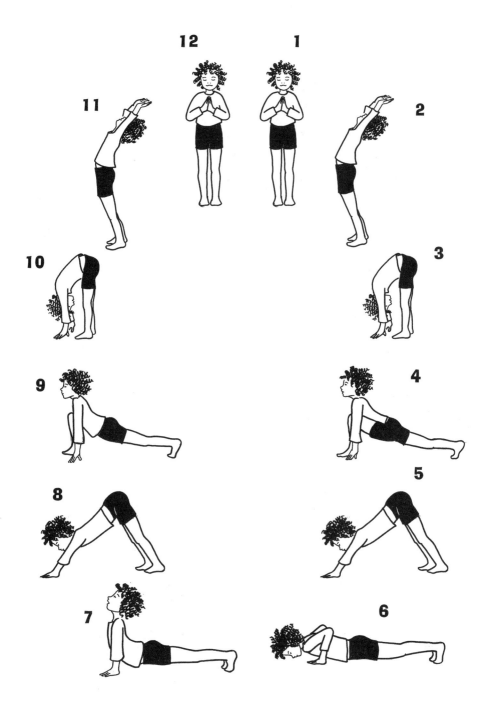

Note: This game can be accompanied by music with Eastern themes or can be done without music. The leader should talk the children through each movement as they do the sun salutation until they have a total body memory of the series of movements.

Imitating Animals

The next section describes a number of yoga postures that are named after animals—with good reason. Children have fun roaring like a lion, flying like a bird, or stretching themselves like a cat.

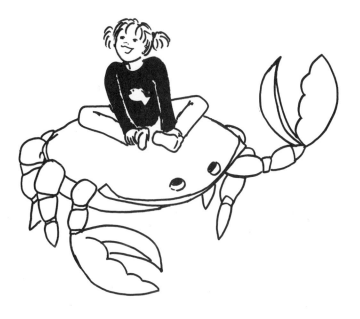

7

Downward-Facing Dog

Most children love dogs. The animals are friendly and playful. Dogs also know how to stretch to recharge their energy. Invite children to stretch like a dog.

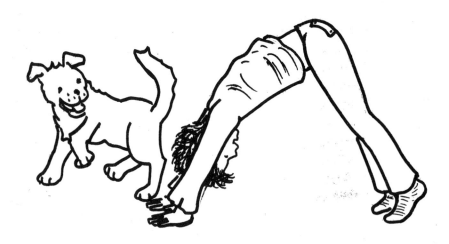

Instructions: Have the children get down on their hands and knees. Tell them to spread their fingers and bend their toes against the ground. As they inhale, they should lift their bodies and push their bottoms in the air. Their feet should now be flat on the floor, and they should be looking at their navels. They should lengthen their spines as much as possible and let their heads hang low to the floor. Next, have them gently breathe in and out and pause for a moment. Then, have them return to the original position. Repeat the exercise two more times.

Cow's Head

Ask the children what they know about cows. What do cows eat? Have they ever watched a cow grazing contentedly? A cow moves its head in a certain way as it eats. Invite children to practice moving like a cow.

Instructions: Have the children sit on the floor. They should slide their right legs along the outside of their left legs. Next, have them sit down on their left heels. As they inhale, instruct them to raise both arms. Then, as they exhale, they should place their right hands on their right shoulders and put their left hands on their lower backs. Now, tell them to slide their right hands downward and their left hands upward. Then the children should try clasping their hands together. Once the hands are clasped (or moved as close together as possible), have them breathe in and out gently and then have them pause for a moment. Then have them return to the starting position. The children should repeat the exercise using the opposite legs and arms.

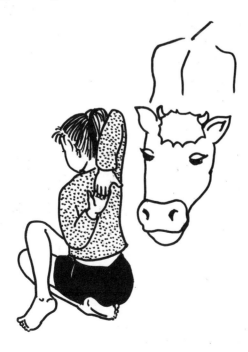

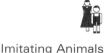
Eagle

The eagle is one of the largest and most impressive birds in the world. Ask children to describe an eagle. Is it beautiful? Strong? Tell them to close their eyes and imagine an eagle standing on a high rock, watching over a valley. Now invite the children to practice moving like an eagle.

Instructions

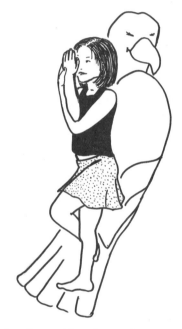

- In the starting position, have the children stand with their feet together and their arms by their sides.
- Next, have the children bend their left legs at the knee. Ask them to elevate the lower part of their left legs and then wrap their left feet/ankles around their right legs, bending their right legs slightly. The backs of their left thighs will then be resting on the fronts of their right thighs.
- Then have the children extend their arms in front of them, parallel to the floor, and cross their right arms over their left arms. They should then bend their arms at the elbows in such a way so that the palms of their hands are facing and their fingers are pointing upward. Have them inhale deeply, making themselves as tall as they can.
- Now tell the children to breathe normally and pause for a moment. They should then return again to the starting position.
- Have the children repeat the exercise using the opposite arms and legs.

Turtle

Turtles can pull themselves back into their shells. Ask: "Try and see if you can pull yourself into your shell and be totally alone and quiet."

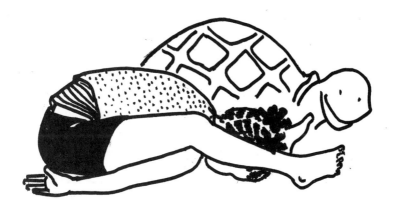

Instructions: Guide the children as follows: *Sit up straight. Stretch your legs in front of you in a V shape. Breathe in, raising your arms. Now breathe out, lowering your arms and head to the ground. Next, move your arms backward and under your thighs. Place them on the floor with your palms facing upward. Close your eyes and stay in this position. Pause for a minute. Then slowly move back into a sitting position.*

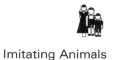

11

Camel

The camel is a common form of transport in the desert. Ask children to imagine that they are riding a camel over warm desert sands. Now tell them they will be doing the camel pose.

Instructions: Tell the children: *Kneel down, keeping your body up straight. Stretch out your arms at shoulder level. Lower your arms slowly and rest your hands on your ankles. As you inhale, bend your neck slowly and gently backward. Push your tummy forward gently. Breathe out, raising your head again. Repeat the exercise two more times and rest.*

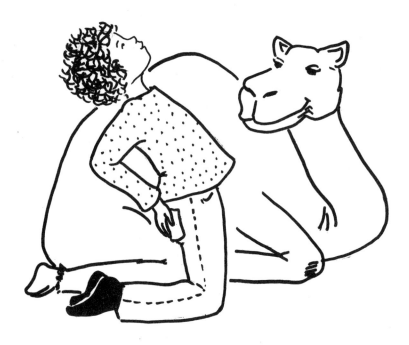

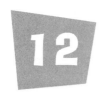

Bird

Tell children to think of birds flying in the air. Ask: "What can birds do that people can't do? Wouldn't it be wonderful to be as free as a bird and fly in the air?" Then, tell them they are going to do the bird posture.

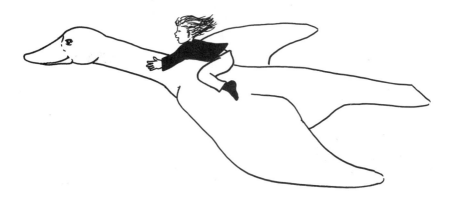

Instructions: Guide the children as follows: *Stand up straight with your feet together. Inhale, raising your arms sideways to shoulder height, with your palms facing downward. As you breathe out, bring your arms down. At the same time, bend your knees. Breathe in and stand up straight again. Repeat this exercise ten times.*

Horse

Horses are noble animals that are frequently admired by children. Ask children to imagine a horse running and jumping. Now tell them that they can show how they can jump like a horse, too.

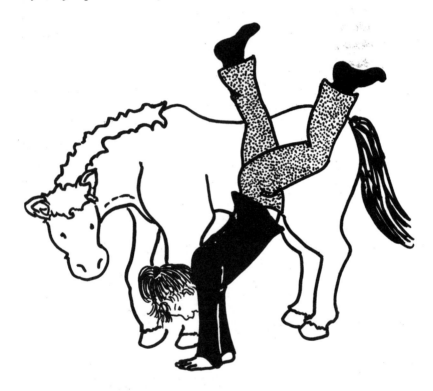

Instructions: Make sure the children have enough space. Tell them to be careful not to kick anyone. Guide them as follows: *Bend over forward with hands flat on the floor. Bend your knees a little. Swing your right foot up and back. As it touches the ground, swing the left foot up. Repeat this ten times.*

Note: This exercise may require supervision. If you are working with a large group, divide the participants into pairs and have one partner do the exercise while the other one watches and makes sure their partner is safe and is no danger of kicking someone else.

From Caterpillar to Butterfly

Every butterfly spends a lot of time being a roly-poly caterpillar. To turn into a butterfly, the caterpillar first spins a cocoon around itself. It transforms into a butterfly inside the cocoon. Then when it is ready, it emerges from the cocoon as a colorful butterfly.

Instructions: Tell the children: *Now it is your turn to show how you can come out of a cocoon as a beautiful butterfly.*

First, invite them to do the caterpillar shuffle.

Have the children bend forward and place their hands on the floor in front of them. They should jump forward with their feet and then move their hands forward and jump forward with their feet again. Have the children repeat the hopping several times.

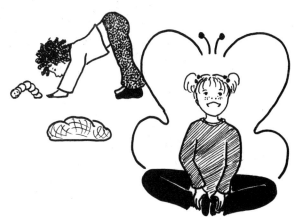

It is now time for the caterpillar to change into a butterfly. Instruct the children as follows:

The caterpillar gets tired and has to lie down. Make yourself very small. Imagine you are sleeping in your cocoon. (Pause for a moment.) *The caterpillar pupates and transforms into a beautiful butterfly. Break out of your cocoon. Now straighten your wings and fly around the room.*

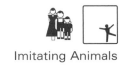
15

Frog

Frogs love to jump in the air, but they can also sit still for a very long time. Children can pretend to jump like frogs from one lily pad to the next on the pond.

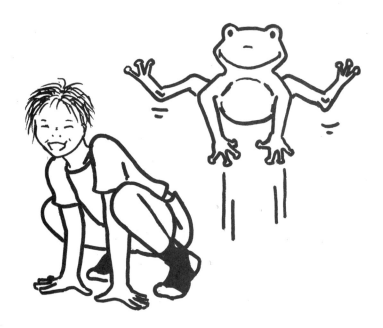

Instructions: Tell the children to crouch down with their legs placed a bit apart. Next, have them place their hands flat on the floor in front of them. Explain to them that they should breathe in as they hop up and then breathe out again as they come down. Have them repeat the exercise several times.

Mouse

Mice are often looking for small places in which to hide from cats and owls. If children have been doing an energetic exercise, it's nice to change the pace a bit. They can relax by going into their "mouse hole."

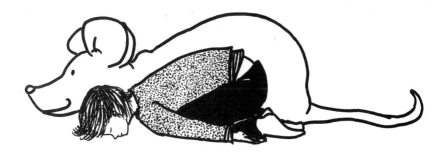

Instructions: Tell the children to kneel with their knees pressed together. Then have them lean forward until their foreheads are on the ground. At this point, have the children place their arms on the floor close to their bodies. Explain that now they're in their mouse holes.

Have the children stay still in their mouse hole for a few minutes. Then, tell them to slowly sit up again.

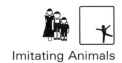

Owl

Owls see and hear much better than people do. Owls hear small prey, such as rabbits or mice, from far away. This makes them very good hunters. They can even turn their heads almost full circle.

Instructions: Invite children to imagine being an owl. Tell them: *Crouch down with your knees together. Put your arms behind your back and clasp your fingers together. Open your eyes very wide. Turn your head as far around as you can. Look over your shoulder as if you are watching for prey. Pretend you see a rabbit. Now open your arms wide and stand up. Fly around the room to catch your prey, making "hoo, hoo" sounds like an owl.*

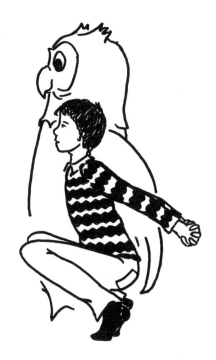

Shark

Sharks are strong and powerful. They swim very fast, and their eyes focus clearly in the dark water. Ask children to imagine that they are sharks. What would they feel like? Now invite the children to move around like a shark.

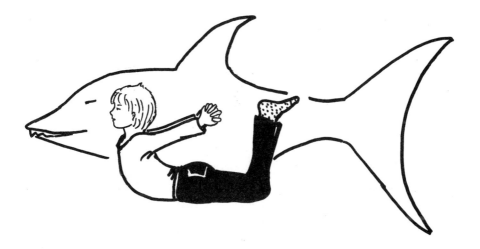

Instructions: Have the children lie on their stomachs. They should bend their legs at the knees and then point their feet at the ceiling to pretend their feet are shark tails. Now tell the children to bring their arms behind them and clasp their fingers together. Next, have them stretch their arms upward to make fins.

Say: *Now you are a shark. Lift your head. Move your tail and fin left and right as if you are swimming in the water.*

Penguin

Children will enjoy waddling around like penguins. Penguins have wings, but they can't fly. They use their wings to help them keep warm.

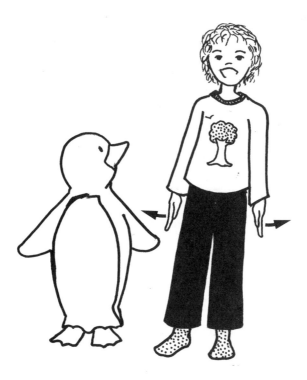

Instructions: You can say: *Penguins live around the South Pole, where all of the land is made of ice. Warm yourself up by flapping your wings.*

Tell the children to stand up straight with their feet slightly apart and their arms by their sides. Keeping their arms straight, ask them to slap their palms against their legs. Have them do this fast and then slow.

Variation: Have the children make shuffling steps around the room as they flap their wings.

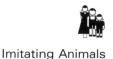
Seal

On land, a seal is clumsy. However, in the water a seal is as graceful as a fish. Ask the children to pretend they are seals. Invite them to roll and slide in the water, feeling free.

Instructions: Have the children lie on their stomachs and stretch their arms out in front of them. Tell them to bring their hands together. Then, have them bring their arms and legs off the ground. They should clap their hands like seals clap their flippers. As the children move, have them make *"onk, onk"* noises like seals.

Variation: Have the children swim away by moving their arms and legs left and right.

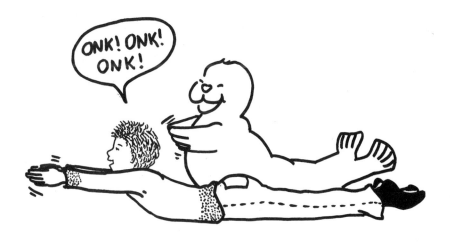

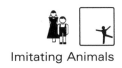
Crab

Crabs are fascinating creatures. They can walk in any direction on land and also in the sea. Invite children to move like crabs.

Instructions: Have the children sit on the floor with their legs stretched out in front of them. Ask them to bend their knees and put their hands flat on the floor behind them with their fingers pointing forward. Then have them lean back and raise their bodies off the ground by standing on their hands and feet.

Tell them: *Imagine you are a crab. Try walking sideways on your hands and feet. Go to the left and then to the right.*

≋ Adventures in the Forest

The games in this section (Games #22–27) describe a series of yoga postures that are performed while a story is being told. Children imagine they are going on an adventure in the forest, where they will experience many different things. They will move around the room and imitate the sounds of the animals they meet.

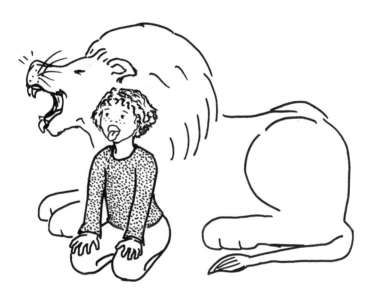

22

Tree

Ask the children to close their eyes and listen to you tell a story. Say: *Imagine you are walking in a forest. A big, leafy tree attracts your attention. You stand up straight and as still as that tree.*

Have the children assume the posture of a tree. They should bend their right knees slightly and then grab their left ankles with their left hands. Next, have the children place their left feet against the insides of their right knees and straighten their legs. They should then put their hands together in front of their chests. If they have trouble balancing, they should do this close to a wall and use the wall to help them get into the posture.

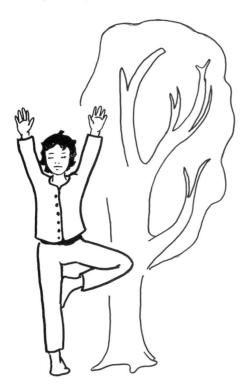

Say: *Your hands are like the tree's leaves, and your arms are like the tree's branches. Raise your hands above your head and open your arms, reaching for the sky.*

Have the children stay still in this position for a moment. Then have them repeat the exercise using the other leg.

Adventures in the Forest

Cobra

The cobra is the next animal the children will encounter on their journey. Continue the story by saying: *You leave your friend the tree and continue to walk down the forest path. You see an old log on the ground, and you hear something coming from behind the log. As you walk closer to investigate, you see a group of cobras hiding behind the log. They greet you with hisses.*

Tell the children to assume the cobra posture. First, they should lie on their stomachs with their legs together. Then, tell them to place their hands flat on the floor next to their chests and look down. Next, have them push up with their arms until the upper parts of their bodies come off the ground and their arms are straight. As children move, tell them to *"hissssss"* like a snake as they look around at each other. Then have the children lie down again. They should repeat the movement two more times.

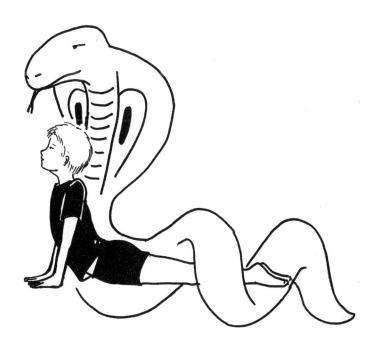

Elephant

The forest adventure continues. Say: *You decide not to spend too much time by the snakes so you continue walking. After a while, you become thirsty and decide to look for water. You hear the noise of running water and make your way toward the river. When you get to the riverbank, you see a herd of elephants drinking.*

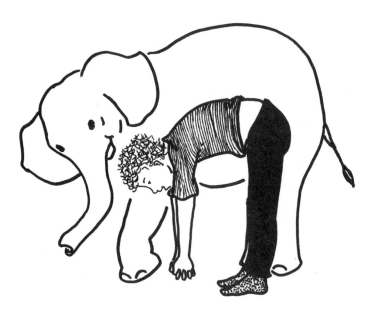

Ask children to imagine that they are big, powerful elephants. Have the children bend forward and straighten their legs. Next, they should clasp their fingers and let their arms hang in front of them like an elephant's trunk. As they breathe in, have them raise their trunks in the air. They should stretch in order to raise their trunks as high as they can. Now, have the children breathe out and bend again. They should repeat the movement five times.

Ape

Continue telling the story: *You walk along the riverbank in search of a place to take a drink. All around you are apes playing in the trees. When the coast is clear, they come down from the trees and play on the ground. They jump all over the place, having lots of fun. The male apes run back and forth, banging their fists on their chests and saying, "oo oo oo." The females swing their arms forward and say, "aah aah aah."*

Have the children bend forward with their legs straight and place their hands on the floor. They should then jump by bringing their hands and feet off the floor together, slightly bending their knees as they land. As they jump, tell the children to make ape sounds. They should repeat the jumps ten times.

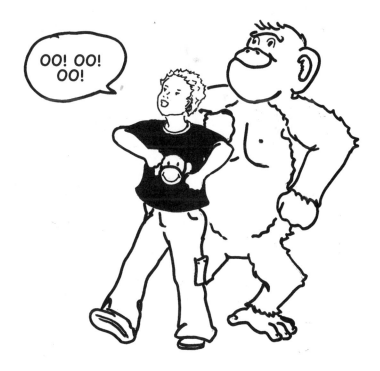

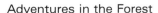
Lion

The adventure continues: *Suddenly the roaring of a lion scares you. The lion is king of the jungle. Make yourself feel as strong as a lion, and roar as hard as you can.*

Kneel down and rest your bottom on your heels. Put your hands on your knees and let your head hang down. As you breathe in, bring your head up. Now open your eyes wide, stick out your tongue and roar "grrrr" as loud as you can.

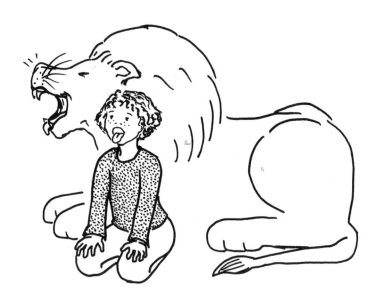

Bear

The story continues: *You get out of the lion's way and continue walking down the forest path. Around a corner, you come across a group of bears taking a walk.*

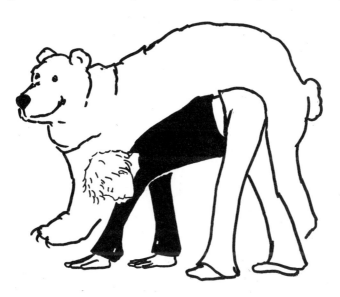

Tell the children to get on their hands and knees and then straighten their legs. Then, have them move around the room by bringing their right hands and right feet forward, then their left hands and left feet.

It's now time for the story to end. Say: *After walking for a long time, the bear gets tired and takes a rest. Lie on the ground and close your eyes. Think about your journey through the forest.* (Pause for a few minutes.) *Then open your eyes.*

⟿ Exercises with a Partner

The following exercises (Games #28–31) are designed for two children working together. For many of the exercises, it might be best to pair children of similar size and strength as partners.

These exercises also offer an opportunity to focus on healthy communication. The children learn to work together to reach a common goal. Before beginning any partner exercise, remind children to be respectful of each other and each other's physical limits. Ask them to be gentle, and remind them to do the movements at a speed that will be comfortable for both of them.

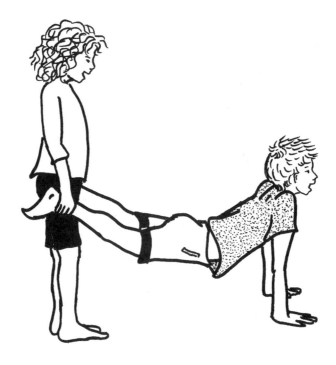

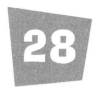

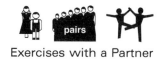

Exercises with a Partner

Bending Sideways

Bending can increase flexibility and improve range of motion in joints. It can even enhance balance. Bending is also an easy exercise that two children can help each other do. Before they begin, instruct the children to pick which side they are going to bend first.

Instructions: Have both children stand straight with their backs to each other, and have them hold each other's hands. Then, as they breathe in, tell the children to raise their clasped hands together and stretch their arms as high as they can. As they breathe out, they should bend over to the previously agreed-upon side. As they breathe in, they should stand straight again. Then, have them repeat the bending movement on their other side. Children should do this exercise twice on each side.

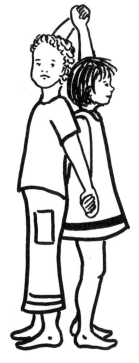

Up and Down

This exercise builds muscle strength in the legs. Alone, a child would be unable to complete this exercise. Together, however, the children can combine their strength to achieve results.

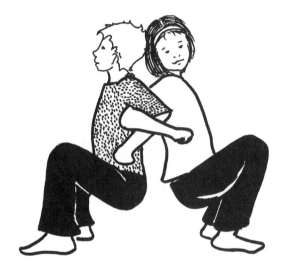

Instructions: Ask the children to sit on the floor back to back, and have them link arms at the elbows. Tell them to bend their knees in such a way so that their feet are firmly planted on the floor. At the count of three, have them push up against each other until they raise their bottoms off the floor. Then they should push down again until they are once again seated. Children should repeat this exercise three times.

Dangling

This exercise builds trust while it stretches the muscles of the back.

Instructions: Have the children stand straight, with their toes touching and firmly holding one another's hands, and then have them look each other in the eyes. Tell the children to gently lean backward as they bend their knees, and to hold each other's hands to help them keep their balance. They should see how close they can come to the floor without losing balance. Then, have them return to a standing position. Children should repeat this exercise five times.

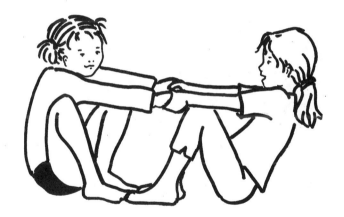

Wheelbarrow

This exercise is an enjoyable way to improve coordination and upper-arm strength.

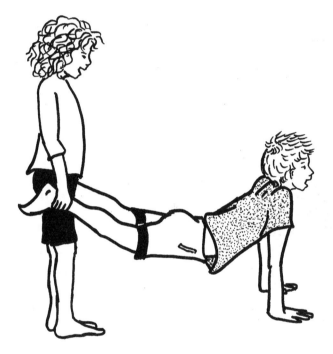

Instructions: Tell one child (A) to lie on the ground with his hands flat on the floor in front of him. His partner (B) should then take hold of A's feet. Have A straighten his arms and push his body off the floor so he can walk on his hands. B should then steer A around the room, holding his feet like the handles of a wheelbarrow. After going round the room once, have the partners switch places.

Yoga Games

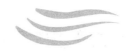

Yoga games are a fun way to promote healthy activity. Movement increases the heart rate and improves circulation throughout the body. Using muscles improves strength, endurance, and flexibility.

Playing together is healthy and also enhances children's social skills. Group play helps children communicate their ideas and wishes. In turn, it exposes them to other people's viewpoints and ideas. An open exchange of thoughts can help children learn to consider each other, to trust each other, and to take responsibility for their actions. As a result, they derive more enjoyment and better results from working together.

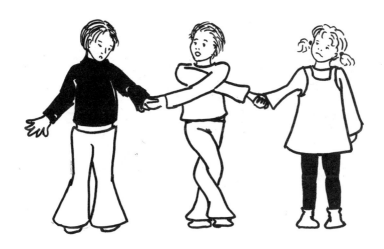

Living Tunnel

Have the children line up side-by-side and get down on their hands and knees. Doing forms a human tunnel. Tell the child at the end of the line to crawl through the tunnel and join the line again at the front. Have all the children do this in turn until everyone has had a chance to crawl through the tunnel.

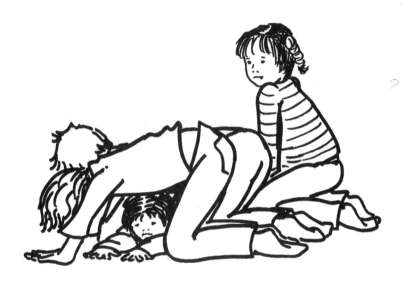

Walking Numbers

Ask one child to think of a number between one and nine. Then have her walk around in an effort to create a picture of the number by the way she moves. The other children should follow her and try to guess what the number is. The child who guesses correctly can think of the next number.

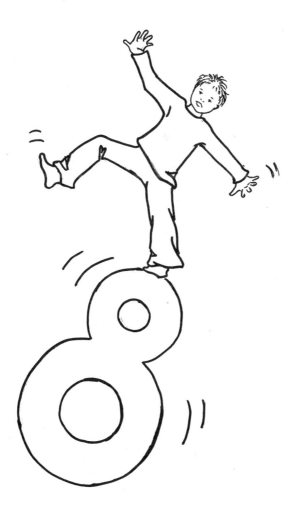

Guessing Letters

Ask one child to think of a letter. He should then use his body to demonstrate the letter to the other children. It doesn't matter if he is lying down or standing up. The other children have to guess which letter it is.

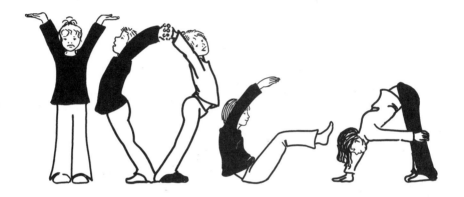

Variation: Have the children work in pairs or small groups instead of in a large group. Players have to think of a word and demonstrate it to the rest of the children. The children in the other groups then have to guess which word is being represented.

Yoga Games

Getting Knotted

Have children stand in a line holding hands. Then, have them form a knot by stepping over and under each other's hands until no one can move any more. Once that is accomplished, have them undo the knot again without letting go of anyone's hands.

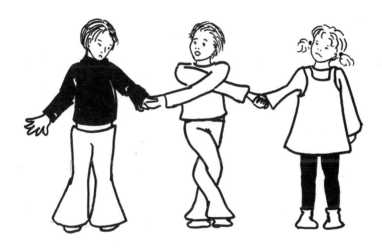

Freezing and Melting

Ask the children to form a circle and stand perfectly still, as if they are frozen. When you are ready, call the name of some part of the body. Each player should then allow this part to "thaw" and move.

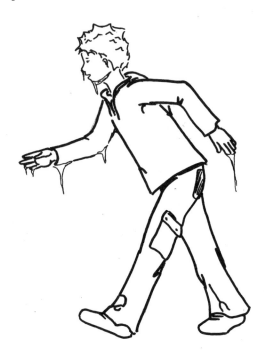

Instruct children as follows: *Stand up straight with your eyes closed. Very slowly your body begins to thaw. First the fingers,... (pause) your arms,... (pause) your torso,... (pause) your legs,... (pause) and your head. Once the whole body is defrosted, start moving around the room.*

Variation: Reverse the procedure and let the children's bodies freeze, bit by bit.

Passing the Balloon

Props: One or more balloons

Have the children sit in a circle with their legs stretched out in front of them. Toss a balloon into the circle, and tell the children that they must use their feet to pass the balloon to the person sitting on their right. Remind them to be gentle so the balloon doesn't pop.

Variation: Make this game even more fun by having two or three balloons going around the circle.

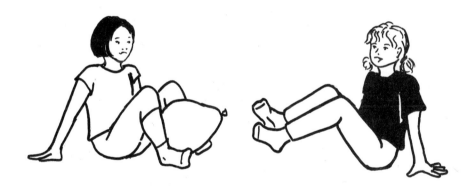

Breathing Exercises

Children can train their breathing to positively impact health. The yoga breathing exercises in the following section can help channel energy and reduce stress and tension.

Most children aren't usually conscious of their breathing. These breathing exercises will help them relax and make them conscious of the force of their breathing. They'll learn to breathe deeply, which is good for their lungs.

Before beginning a breathing exercise, instruct children to inhale through their nose as much as possible. This ensures that the air is warmed and the hairs in the nose filter any dust.

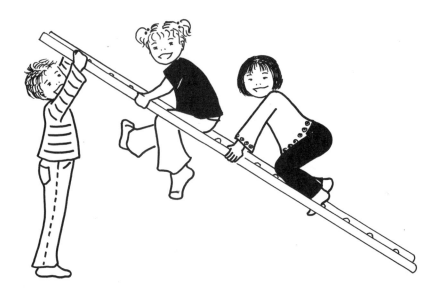

38

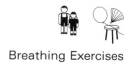
Teddy Breathing

Props: A teddy bear or other stuffed animal

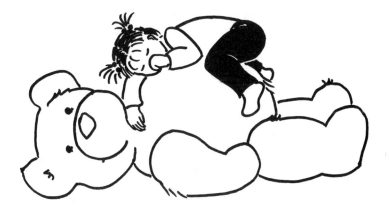

Most children will understand the best way to breathe if they can see what they are doing. Have the children put a teddy bear or other stuffed animal on their stomachs. Tell them to watch the toys as they breathe.

Say: *Lie on your back with your eyes closed. Try to make the toy on your stomach move up and down with your breath. Breathe in and out just as you normally do.*

Balloon Breathing

This exercise enables children to become conscious of their breathing because it allows them to focus on the way in which the air flows in through the nose and out again. Instruct the children as follows: *Sit up straight with your legs crossed and close your eyes. Put your hands on your stomach and concentrate on your breathing. Feel how your stomach fills up as you breathe in. Feel how it goes down as you breathe out. Imagine a balloon inside your stomach that fills itself with air when you inhale and then empties itself of air when you exhale. As you breathe, try to feel the balloon with your hands. Do this for about one minute.*

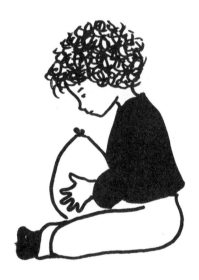

The Breathing Ladder

This exercise requires at least three children and one adult. You, the adult, should closely monitor the exercise to be sure that everyone assumes the correct position.

Instructions: Have the first child lie on his back with his legs outstretched and his arms by his sides. Then, have the next child lie down on her back oriented in such a way so that she can gently put her head on the stomach of the first child. Other children should then join the "ladder" in the same way. Ask the children to feel and listen to see if the whole ladder can breathe together.

Breathing with Sounds

Sounds help emphasize the breathing process.

Instructions: Have the children sit cross-legged with their hands in their laps. Pick a sound that you want the group to hear and then make it. Ask the children to inhale deeply. As they exhale, have them mimic the sound you made. Try the exercise again with a different sound.

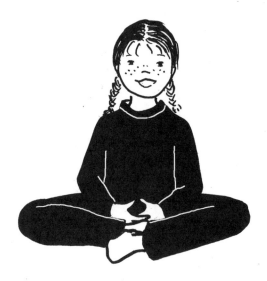

Note: The following sounds work well with this exercise: *HA, AH, O, OO, MMM, ZZZ.* You can also use animal noises.

Concentration and Meditation

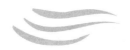

Yoga principles can help children focus. Through the practice of meditation and concentration, children can learn to keep their attention on one thing. They can train themselves to master their thoughts. Part of this process is learning to decide for themselves whether they want to think about something now or later.

Encourage children to communicate what things distract them. This acknowledgement makes them more aware and in control of their senses. If they hear a sound outside, they can call that "hearing." If they are tempted look at something, they can call that "seeing."

Another way to help children concentrate is to have them focus their attention on everyday things. For example, during meals children could focus on chewing and tasting. At other times, they could concentrate on reading or watching television.

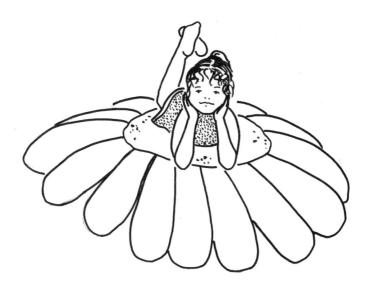

Correct Posture

Good posture is very important for meditation. Encourage children to sit up straight and walk tall. These postures create a feeling of power and make it possible to breathe more deeply.

Instructions: Guide the children as follows: *Sit cross-legged with your hands in your lap. Imagine that your spine is the stem of a flower, sucking water from the ground. Water flows better up a straight stem than a bent one; the same applies to your spine. Sit up straight, and follow your breathing in and out.*

After one to five minutes, have the children open their eyes again.

Sitting Still and Counting

This exercise will help children learn to detach from distractions.

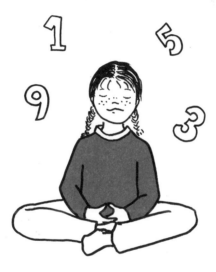

Instructions: Ask the children to sit up straight with their legs crossed and their hands in their laps. Then, have them join their thumbs and forefingers together to make a circle.

Now the leader says: *Close your eyes and breathe gently (pause). Listen to the sounds around you (pause). Detach yourself from the sounds, and begin slowly counting from one to ten. Each time another thought comes into your mind, stop counting and begin again at one. If you manage to reach ten, use the same method to count down again to one.*

After one to five minutes, have the children open their eyes again.

Watching the Clock

Watching the Clock is designed to help children focus.

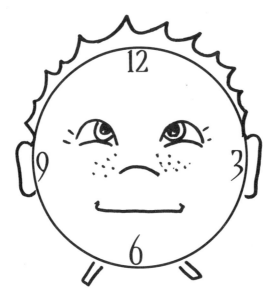

Instructions: Ask the children to sit up straight with their legs crossed. Guide them as follows: *Imagine that you have a clock painted on your face. Look upward as much as you can. Focus on the point in the middle of your forehead where the twelve would be on a clock face. Hold this position for a count of five. Now turn your eyes to the one position on the clock face. Pause for a moment. Next, turn your eyes to the two position and so on until you are back at the twelve.*

Children should then repeat the exercise in a counterclockwise direction.

Walking

A simple way to bring conscious action into daily life is to concentrate on the experience of walking.

Instructions: Tell the children: *Walk slowly around the room. Concentrate your attention on your feet. Be conscious of placing your foot on the floor. Observe how it feels when your foot makes contact with the ground. How does the weight move? How does it lift from the ground again? Keep your attention only on the act of walking. Carefully observe every step and how it feels.*

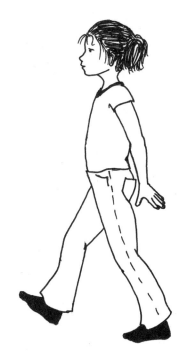

Flower Meditation

Props: One flower per child

Too often people take things in the natural world for granted. This exercise uses a simple flower to awaken and focus the senses.

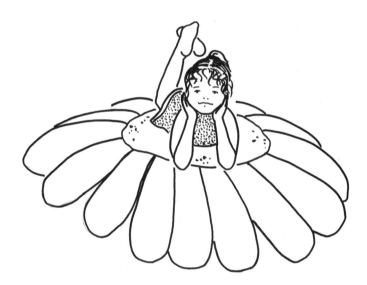

Instructions: Give each child a flower. Instruct the children as follows: *Sit up straight with your legs crossed. Examine your flower. How does it feel? How does it smell? Now place the flower on the floor in front of you. Close your eyes and breathe gently. Try to bring the flower into your mind. Can you see the colors? Can you recall the smell? Can you sense how it felt?*

Pause for several minutes. Then tell them to open their eyes. Encourage the children to talk about their experiences.

Balloon Meditation

Becoming aware of their thoughts and learning how to detach from them is the focus of this exercise.

Instructions: Ask the children to sit up straight with their legs crossed and their hands in their laps. Then, have them join their thumbs and forefingers together to make a circle.

Guide them as follows: *Imagine you are blowing up a balloon, and it is getting bigger each time you breathe out.* (Pause for a moment.) *When the balloon is big enough, put all your busy thoughts inside it.* (Pause for a moment.) *Tie a knot in the balloon and blow it high into the air.*

After a few minutes, tell the children they can open their eyes. Ask them to share their experiences. What thoughts did they put in their balloon? What color was their balloon? How high did it fly when they blew it away? Did they find the exercise easy or difficult?

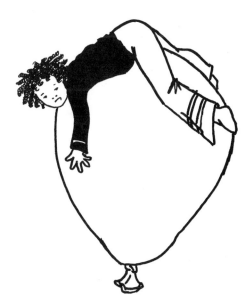

Exercising the Senses

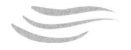

This section contains exercises designed to help children focus their senses. The senses are one of the main ways people connect to the world around them. By becoming conscious of their senses, children can better experience their environment.

All of a person's senses are directed outward. If someone smells, hears, tastes, feels, or sees something, the attention is drawn in that direction. For this reason, a person's senses can be very distracting. Yet if focused properly, they can bring a great deal of pleasure.

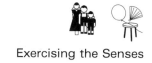

Smelling

Props: A variety of fragrant materials, such as grass, perfume, spices, and flowers

Tell the children to sit in a circle with their eyes closed. Then, pass a basket or container with one fragrant item in it under each child's nose. Ask the children to raise their hand if they know what the item is. Call on one of the children who thinks she knows the answer and have her tell the others what she thinks it is, and then see if the other children agree. Then have the children open their eyes and look at the item. You can repeat this exercise with a variety of different fragrances.

Examples

- Flowers
- Grass
- Earth
- Charcoal
- Perfume
- Spices
- Sweets
- Cookies
- Fruit

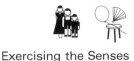

Hearing

Props: A recording of a variety of everyday sounds, such as birds, airplanes, and cars

Ask the children to sit in a circle. Play the sound recording, stopping after each sound. Have the children try to guess what each sound is.

Examples

- Everyday sounds—birds, airplanes, cars, a person walking up some stairs, etc.
- Bells
- Rain stick
- Drum

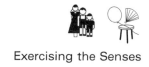

Tasting

Props: A variety of foods with distinct tastes

Tell the children sit in a circle with their eyes closed. Distribute one food at a time and have everyone taste it. Have the children try to guess what each food is. Pause after each food.

Examples

- Sweet (sugar, raisins, or sweets)
- Sour (berries, lemons, or sour apples)
- Salt (salt licorice or sea salt)
- Bitter (coffee or basil)

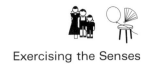

Feeling

Props: A variety of objects with varying forms, shapes, and weights

Have the children sit in a circle with their eyes closed. Pass around one of the objects, and have every player take a turn feeling the form, shape, and weight of each object. After the object has been passed to every child, have them try to guess what the object is. Then pause and repeat the exercise until every object has been passed around the circle.

Examples

- Cotton wool
- Sandpaper
- Shells
- Pebbles
- Onion
- Potato
- Tennis ball
- Corrugated cardboard

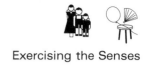

Seeing

Props: A variety of objects of different colors and sizes

Tell the children to sit in a circle with their eyes closed. Place a variety of objects in the center of the circle. Once you have done so, have the children open their eyes and look at each object carefully. After a certain period of time, have them close their eyes again. Once all of the children's eyes are shut, remove one object and tell the children to open their eyes again. The children then have to guess which object has been removed.

Examples
- Feather
- Soft toy
- Ball
- Seashell
- Fruit
- Flower
- Book

Chakra Exercises

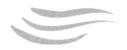

The yoga exercises in this section are designed to have a good effect on the body's chakras. A chakra is a spiritual energy center inside the body. The seven main chakras are situated along the spine at the coccyx, sacrum, navel, heart, throat, forehead, and crown. Each chakra represents a different type of energy and state of mind, which everyone experiences in his or her own way. Each chakra also has its own color, and together they form a rainbow.

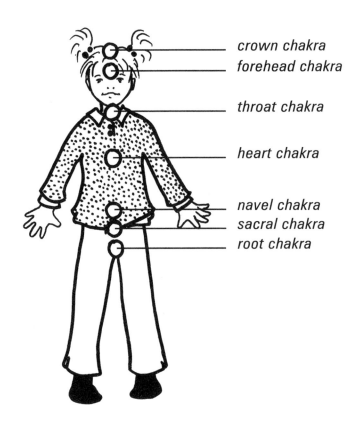

crown chakra
forehead chakra

throat chakra

heart chakra

navel chakra
sacral chakra
root chakra

⁓ Root Chakra

The first chakra is located in the coccyx (perineum), which is situated at the base of the spine. It is associated with the color red. The following two games help stimulate this energy center.

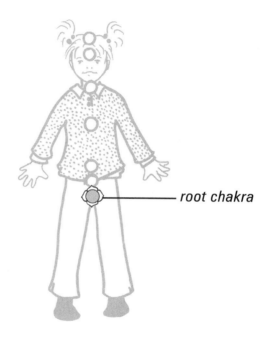

root chakra

Root Chakra

Bouncing

Children can open the root chakra by bouncing gently on their bottoms.

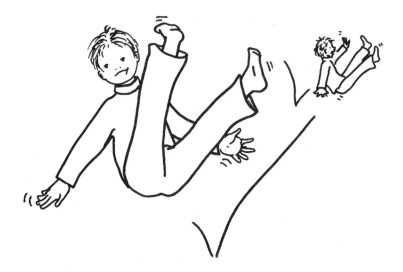

Instructions: Tell them: *Sit up straight with your legs stretched in front of you. Support yourself by putting your hands on the floor behind you with your fingers pointing forward. Lift yourself up and bounce your bottom on the floor ten times.*

Root Chakra

Stomping

Stomping on the ground with both feet is a great way for children to ground themselves. Have the children stand up straight and stomp on the ground, one foot after the other—left, right, left, right.

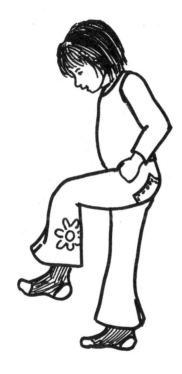

Variation: Play African drum music and get the children to move around the room in time with the drums.

≋ Sacral Chakra

The second chakra is situated at the bottom of the torso at the sacrum and is associated with the color orange. The following exercises help stimulate this energy center.

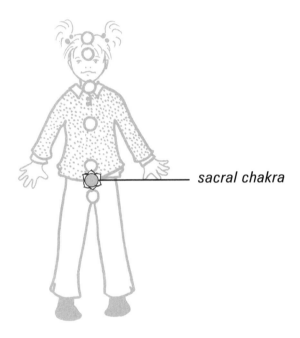

sacral chakra

55

Sacral Chakra

Concave
and Convex

This exercise is also called "The Cat." When a cat is angry, it arches its back. Invite the children to stretch like a cat.

Instructions: Tell them: *Get down on your hands and knees. As you breathe in, sway your back by dropping your tummy toward the floor and bringing your head up. As you breathe out, arch your back and let your head hang down. Repeat the exercise several times in your own rhythm.*

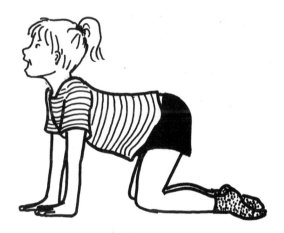

Variation: As they breathe out, have the children say "meow" or have them hiss like a frightened cat.

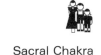

56

Sacral Chakra

Raising the Hips

Have the children lie on their backs with their knees bent and their feet flat on the floor. As they breathe in, tell them to lift their hips toward the ceiling. As they breathe out, tell them to lower their hips to the starting position.

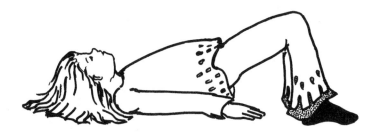

Repeat the exercise several times. Let each child follow his or her own rhythm.

≋ Navel Chakra

The third chakra is the navel chakra, and it is situated behind the navel. It is associated with the color yellow. The following exercises help stimulate this energy center.

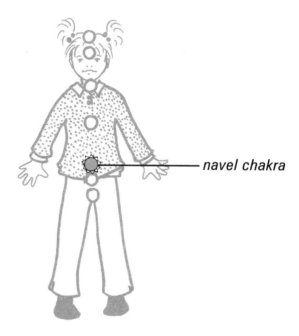

navel chakra

Jumping

The navel chakra represents energy and warmth. Let the children see for themselves how warm they get when they jump.

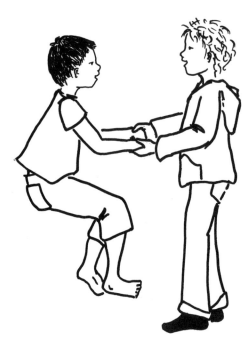

Instructions: Divide the group into pairs. Tell the partners to stand facing one other, holding hands. Each child then takes a turn jumping as high as possible, using their partner's hands as a support. After they have each taken a turn, tell the first child to jump ten times without stopping and then rest for a moment. Now the partner takes a turn jumping.

Pressing the Navel

The navel is an important part of the body. This exercise makes children more aware of their navel.

Instructions: Have the children stand up straight with their fingertips placed around their navel. Tell them: *Concentrate on your breathing. As you breathe out, press your navel gently. Breathe in, and let your fingers release the pressure. Close*

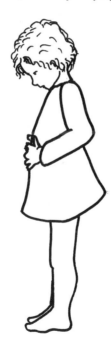

your eyes so you can concentrate on the exercise better and feel what is happening. Repeat the exercise ten times in your own rhythm.

≋ Heart Chakra

The fourth chakra is the heart chakra. It is situated just behind the heart and is associated with the color green. The following exercises help stimulate this energy center.

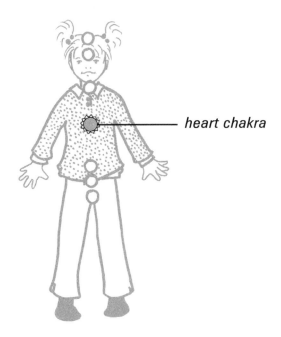

heart chakra

Heart Chakra

Circles

This exercise raises the heart rate and increases blood flow through the body.

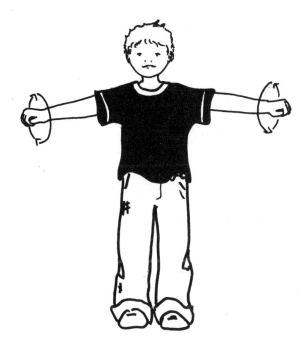

Instructions: Have the children stand up straight with their arms stretched sideways at shoulder height. They should also make fists.

Once in this position, have the children make small forward circles with their arms that should steadily get bigger. When the circles reach their maximum size, tell the children to start making backward circles with their arms that should get smaller and smaller. When the exercise is finished, have the children drop their arms and shake them until they feel loose.

Heart Chakra

Up and Down

This exercise is good to use after a more active one. It can be relaxing and helps children focus.

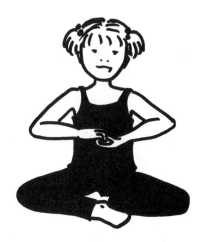

Instructions: Tell them: *Sit up straight with your legs crossed. Bring your hands level with your heart, clasp your fingers, and pull your elbows apart gently. In time with your breathing, raise and lower your hands. When you have finished, shake your arms and shoulders until they feel loose again.*

≋ Throat Chakra

The fifth chakra is the throat chakra. It is situated in the throat and is associated with the color blue. The following exercises help stimulate this energy center.

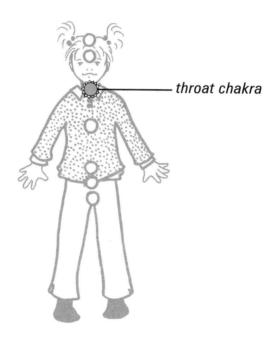

throat chakra

Backward and Forward

This exercise gives children the opportunity to focus on the throat chakra as well as on breathing techniques.

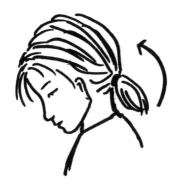

Instructions: Have the children sit up straight with their legs crossed. As they breathe in, tell them to gently lean their heads backward, and as they breathe out, tell them to rest their chins on their chests.

Repeat the exercise several times. Let each child follow his or her own rhythm.

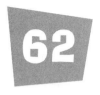

Throat Chakra

From Right to Left

This exercise uses the muscles of the neck.

Instructions: Tell the children to sit up straight with their legs crossed. As they breathe in, have them turn their heads to the right, and as they breathe out, have them bring their heads back to the middle. The next time they breathe in, tell them to turn to the left, and as they breathe out, have them turn back to the middle once again. Ask them to do this without moving their shoulders, so that only their heads move. Instruct children to use a gentle, fluid motion when they turn their heads. They shouldn't force the movement or they could strain their necks.

Repeat the exercise several times.

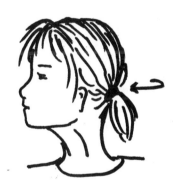

Shoulder to Shoulder

It is important to have the correct posture for this exercise. Make sure children do not hunch their shoulders. Tell them to bring their heads down to the shoulders and not their shoulders up to their heads.

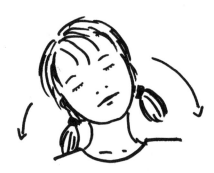

Instructions: Guide them as follows: *Sit up straight with your legs crossed. Breathe in. As you do so, move your right ear down as if you were going to touch it to your right shoulder. As you breathe out, bring your head up straight again. Now breathe in, and bend your head so that your left ear moves as close to your left shoulder as possible. Breathe out and straighten up again. Repeat this exercise several times in your own rhythm.*

Forehead Chakra

The sixth chakra is the forehead chakra. It is situated in the center of the forehead and is associated with the color indigo. The following exercise helps stimulate this energy center.

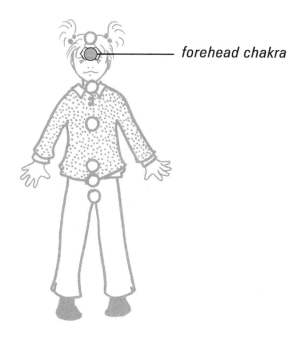

forehead chakra

Elbow Butterflies

Ask the children to imagine colorful butterflies flying around the room. Then invite them to make elbow butterflies.

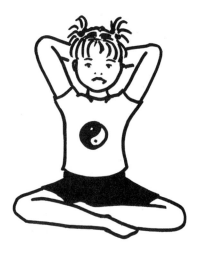

Instructions: Tell them: *Sit up straight with your legs crossed. Place your hands one on top of the other on the back of your head. Point your elbows forward as much as you can until they almost touch each other. As you breathe in, pull your elbows as far back as you can and push your shoulder blades together. Hold your breath for a moment. Then as you breathe out, bring your elbows forward again. Repeat several times in your own rhythm.*

≋ Crown Chakra

The seventh chakra is the crown chakra. It is on the crown of the head and is associated with the color violet. The following exercises help stimulate this energy center.

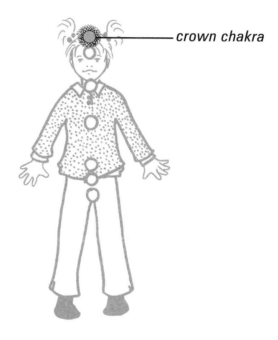

crown chakra

Crown Chakra

Rubbing
the Crown

Ask the children to clear their minds of all distractions before they begin this exercise. Once they have done so, have them sit up straight with their legs crossed and close their eyes, breathing deeply and gently. Then, have them place their right hands on their crowns and rub them softly ten times in a clockwise direction. Tell them that when they are finished, they should remain sitting still and think about the experience. After a couple of minutes, tell the children to open their eyes again.

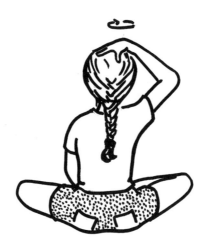

Warm, White Light

This exercise encourages the use of imagination and focus.

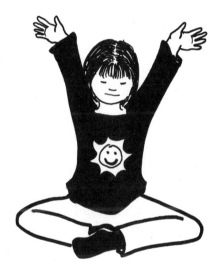

Instructions: Have the children sit up straight with their legs crossed. Tell them to close their eyes and stretch their hands above their heads and to breathe in and out deeply and gently. Now, have them imagine a warm, white light coming into their crowns and flowing down into their bodies. Tell them to feel how warm their body becomes.

Have the children stay sitting for one or two minutes. Then tell them to open their eyes again.

Visualization Exercises

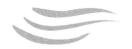

The exercises in this section are designed to help children explore yoga visualization techniques. Visualization exercises help release creative energy and encourage imagination. Children will also practice concentration.

Guided visualizations can take children on wonderful journeys to places of innocence and wonder. For example, the king of the elves guides children on a journey through the woods, showing them the richness of life on Earth. A mermaid guides children on their journey into the ocean to explore the secrets of her underwater kingdom. In an adventure in the clouds, the children meet their guardian angels and take a ride on a cloud. When they go to the Sun, a fire nymph takes them along a sunbeam to get closer to the star.

The stories are enhanced if accompanied by music that uses appropriate natural sounds. When reading a visualization story, pause after each sentence. This allows children the time to create pictures and images of the story in their minds.

When the story is finished, the children can say goodbye to the friends they met on the journey. They should breathe deeply, move their fingers and toes, and then open their eyes again. Afterward, take a little time to talk with the children about their experiences.

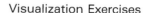
A Walk in the Woods

In this adventure, children will meet an elf who walks with them through the woods. Here is one way to tell the story:

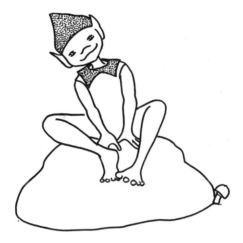

Lie on your back and close your eyes. Breathe softly and deeply. As you breathe, feel your body becoming heavier with each breath. Feel your body pressing more and more on the ground. It is becoming heavier all the time. Imagine you are on a path in beautiful woodland, just after a rainstorm. As you walk, you feel the warm, damp earth beneath your feet. The leaves are green, and the raindrops glisten as they slowly drop to the ground. As they fall, the earth catches and absorbs each one. The sun emerges from behind a cloud and shines through the trees. The birds start singing as they fly from tree to tree. As you walk through the woods, different animals greet you. The woods have come to life again, and even the insects are busy with their work. Further along the path, there is an old tree. You look at it in wonder; it has seen so many lives come and go. Suddenly an elf comes out of the tree and invites you to go with him. He is very friendly and knows all about nature. Anything you want to know about you can ask him. I'm going to leave you here for a while so you can have

a look around. (Pause for two to five minutes.) *Now it's time to say goodbye to your new friend. The elf will bring you home again.*

Encourage the children to share their experiences. Ask them what questions they asked the elf. What did the elf show them in the forest? What kind of animals greeted them as they walked through the woods?

Note: This game is best accompanied by a recording of soothing music or sounds of nature.

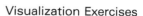
An Ocean Journey

In this adventure, children will meet a mermaid who takes them to her underwater kingdom. Here is one way to tell the story:

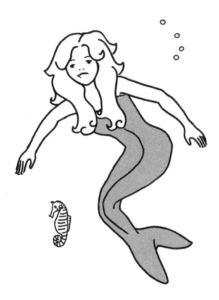

Lie on your back and close your eyes. Breathe gently in and out. Concentrate on your breathing. Now imagine that you are walking along the beach. You feel the warm sand under your feet. Lie down on the lovely warm sand. Let each breath flow over your body like the waves of the ocean. The day is hot, and the sun shines on your body. Your whole body gets warm, and this warmth gives you enough energy to do anything you want. Breathe in and out gently in time with the rhythms of the ocean. Now you hear someone calling your name. It is a dolphin waiting in the sea to take you on an adventure. He knows the sea very well. You feel very safe with the dolphin, and you put your arm around him. When you get into the water, you feel how warm it is. You realize that you can breathe under water as you dive with the dolphin. You notice how very quiet it is under the water. A little further, you come to the coral reef. As the sun glitters through the water, the colors of the reef move and change. You see

schools of fish in every shape, size, and color swimming around the reef. As you go deeper, you meet more dolphins. They play and talk to each other, making soft noises and clicking sounds. They are happy to see you and ask if you want to ride on the back of one of them. This dolphin brings you right down to the ocean floor, which is the kingdom of the mermaids. You can see lots of mermaids swimming in and out of their underwater castles and waving at you. One of them comes and takes you to explore her kingdom with all its secrets. You can stay with her a while so you can enjoy your adventure. (Pause for two to five minutes.) Now it's time to say goodbye. Your dolphin friend comes to take you back to the beach again.

Encourage the children to share their experiences. Ask them what the mermaid showed them. What did the mermaids' castles look like? What were the secrets of the mermaid kingdom? What kind of fish did they see in the reef?

Note: This game is best accompanied by a recording of soothing music or the sounds of the ocean.

Journey to the Clouds

In this adventure, children will meet an angel as they travel through the clouds. Here is one way to tell the story:

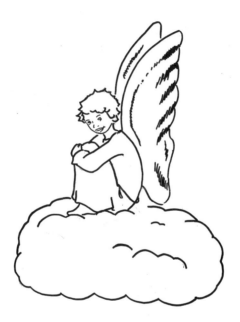

Lie on your back and close your eyes. Breathe in and out softly. Concentrate on your breathing. Feel your body becoming lighter and lighter. Imagine that it's a beautiful day, and that you are lying on your back in the garden. As you look up, you can see lots of clouds in all shapes and sizes, changing all the time. If you look closely, you can see many things in the clouds. Suddenly, you see an angel coming down to take you on a journey in the clouds. It is your guardian angel who is always watching over you. The angel can read your thoughts, so you don't need to speak. If you listen carefully, you can hear her talking to you in your mind. Your guardian angel is ready to take you on a journey to her home in the deep blue sky. On the way, you can

ask her any question you want. You climb onto the cloud with the angel. You leave the earth and float higher and higher on this soft fluffy cloud. On the way, you meet lots of birds and say hello to them. You can see other clouds with children on them. They are also going on journeys with their guardian angels. When you look down, you can see the trees, houses, and people getting smaller and smaller. Now you are high in the air among the clouds. You can walk from one cloud to another. Your guardian angel wants to show you many things, so enjoy your journey. (Pause for two to five minutes). Now it's time to say goodbye. Your guardian angel brings you to a small cloud and you float back down to your garden.

Encourage the children to share their experiences. Ask them what birds they saw as they traveled on the cloud. What did the birds look like? Did they ask their angel any questions? What did their angel look like? What things did their angel show them?

Journey to the Sun

In this adventure, children will meet the Sun King as they travel to the sun. Here is one way to tell the story:

Lie on your back and close your eyes. Breathe in and out gently. Concentrate on your breathing. It is a beautiful day—the sky is blue and the sun is shining. You love the way the sun warms your body. Your head is warm, and so are your arms, your stomach, and your legs. Your whole body is lovely and warm and you are ready to go and greet the sun. Your journey can start at any moment because the fire nymph is coming to take you on a trip. He slowly comes down from the sky, sliding down a sunbeam. He lands in front of you and says hello. He is a funny little man and looks as if he has just stepped out of a fire. Before you go with him, he asks you to protect yourself against the warmth of the sun. You do this by imagining you are wearing a special protective suit. You jump on a sunbeam with him and are on your way to the sun. When you arrive, you see everything around you glittering like gold. In the distance are golden birds flying back and forth. You meet the Sun King and he asks how

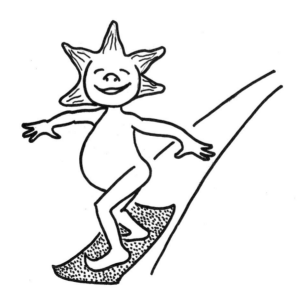

you are. He wants to show you his kingdom and invites you to take a trip in his golden coach. You stay there a little while so you can enjoy this beautiful place. (Pause for two to five minutes.) *Now it's time to say goodbye again. The fire nymph brings you safely home down his sunbeam.*

Encourage the children to share their experiences. What did their protective suit look like? What does the Sun King look like? What did the Sun King's coach look like? What things did they see in the Sun King's kingdom?

Wake-Up Exercises

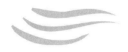

Guided visualizations can be very relaxing, creating an almost sleeplike state. This section contains exercises designed to ease the transition from visualization to increased activity.

The exercises are very well suited to waking up. Children can do the Body Scan (Game #71) to experience the feeling of tensing and relaxing. Once the body is alert and the children are awake again, they can do the Spaghetti Test (Game #76).

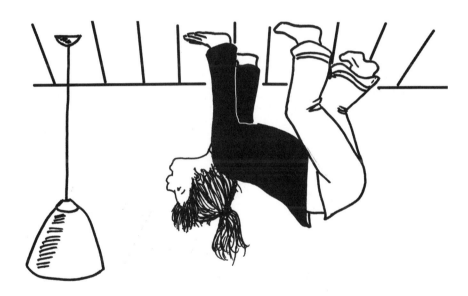

Body Scan

Have the children lie on their backs with their legs straight and their arms by their sides. As they breathe in, tell them to tense a particular body part and hold the tension a moment. Then, as they breathe out, they should relax that part of the body again. After doing that a few times, have the children tense all the different parts of their bodies at the same time and hold the tension a moment. Then, as they breathe out, they should relax their entire bodies. Have the children lie still for a minute to connect to their bodies and feel each sensation.

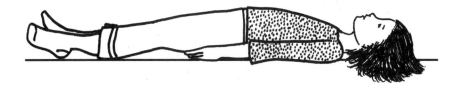

Tip: Suggest that children start by balling up their fists, pointing their toes at the ceiling, scrunching their buttocks, or opening their mouths and eyes wide.

Rubbing Hands and Feet

Each person experiences this exercise differently. Many children have said things like: "It feels like butterflies on my hand," "My hands feel like magnets," "I can feel wispy things between my hands," or "I didn't feel anything."

Instructions: Tell them: *Lie on your back with your legs bent in a way that allows the soles of your feet to touch. Put your hands together, too. Start rubbing your hands and feet together. Continue this for one minute. Now stretch your legs. Close your eyes, and cover them with your hands. Feel the warmth of your hands on your eyes. Lie there and relax for one to two minutes. Now open your eyes.*

Encourage the children to express how this exercise felt to them.

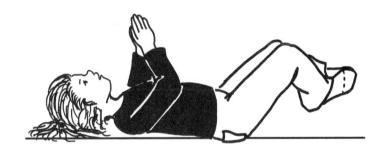

Air Walking

This exercise will raise the heart rate and wake up the body. Instruct children as follows:

Lie on your back with your arms by your sides. As you breathe in, lift your left hand and your right leg. Your palms and the soles of your feet should face the ceiling. As you exhale, let your hand and your leg sink back down to the floor. Breathe in, and raise your right hand and left leg. Repeat this several times.

Back Roll

This exercise will gently rock the body into alertness. Tell them: *Lie on your back. Raise your legs into the air, and cross your feet. Grab your right ankle or shin with your left hand. Grab your left ankle or shin with your right hand. Now, rock back and forth by moving your weight forward and backward.*

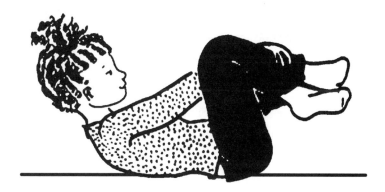

Stretching

A stretch when waking can make the muscles limber and ready for activity. Each child experiences this exercise differently. Children have remarked: "My left side feels taller," "I feel uneven," or "The left side tingles and feels warm."

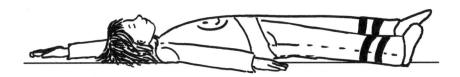

Instructions: Guide them as follows:

Lie on your back with your arms by your sides. As you breathe in, raise your left arm. Bring it back over your head to the floor. Stretch and make your left side as long and tall as you can. Point your toes on your left leg as you stretch this leg and foot as much as you can. As you breathe out, bring your hand back to your side. Relax the left side of your body and your left foot. See how different the left and right sides of your body feel. (Pause for a moment.) *Now do the same exercise with the right arm and the right side of your body.*

Spaghetti Test

Divide the children into pairs. It may be easier for them to relax if you have the children lying down close their eyes. Instruct them as follows:

When you cook spaghetti, you first put long, stiff sticks of pasta into the pan. The spaghetti becomes soft in the hot water. If you try to grab a strand, it will bend in all directions.

Have one child lie on his back and relax his whole body. His partner should then hold one of his hands and gently shake it back and forth like a soft strand of spaghetti. Have the children repeat the test on their partner's other arm. Then have the partners change places.

Note: To be most effective, make sure the child who is lying down doesn't help with the lifting and shaking of his arm. If that happens, the child's muscles will tense, and the arm will not be as soft as spaghetti.

Storytelling

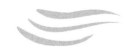

This section contains stories that help children understand the yoga rules for living. The rules help children achieve healthy, balanced lives.

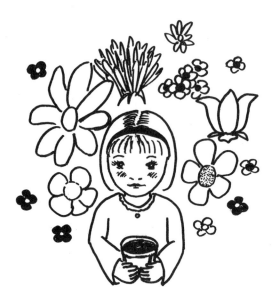

≋ Children and Karma

The principle of karma has a lot in common with yoga rules. People live in a particular family in a particular place with a particular body and spirit, and they learn to make the best of it. According to karma, the way in which a person thinks, does things, or refrains from doing things determines her life and her surroundings. By reading these stories, children come to understand the principle of karma without ever hearing it mentioned by name.

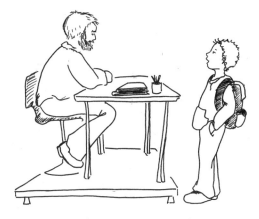

Pupil: "What is karma?"

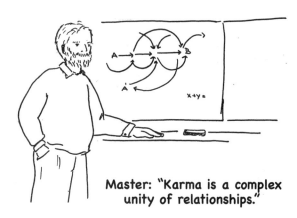

Master: "Karma is a complex unity of relationships."

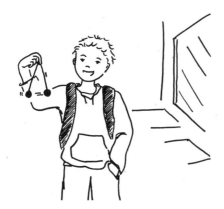

Pupil: "I believe in cause and effect."

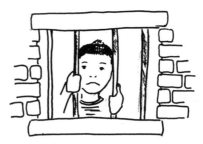

Master: "Look at this young man who
is in prison. He is accused of theft.
Who is guilty–the man who stole, the
friends who set him on the wrong path,
the people who raised him, or the
person who caught him and didn't
prevent him from stealing?"

The Honest Princess

Read the story to the children. Encourage them to share their ideas about the story's meaning afterward.

Long ago there was a prince who was looking for a wife. Because his future wife would later become queen, he had to find an honest young woman. He invited all the young women who would like to marry him to visit the palace.

One beautiful day, all the young women arrived in their most elegant clothes. Each was more beautiful than the one before her, and they were all wearing fabulous jewelry. In fact, they all looked like princesses! They all wanted to impress the prince. Right at the back was a young girl who stood out because she was wearing her everyday clothes. She really wanted to meet the prince because she loved him very much.

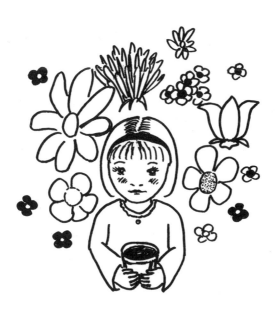

On this lovely summer's day, he did not make a choice from all the beautiful girls. Instead he gave each one a seed. The one who in six months time could bring him the most beautiful flower grown from this seed would become his wife. Each of the girls took her seed and went home.

The girl in the everyday clothes put her seed into a flowerpot with some earth. She cared for it with patience and love. Three months went by, but nothing grew. It seemed that her dream was beyond her reach, but still she didn't give up hope. She was determined. After six months, she returned to the palace with her flowerpot.

When the prince came in, he looked carefully into all the flowerpots the girls had brought with them. They all had the most beautiful flowers, each more lovely than the one before. After the prince had looked at all the flowers, he pointed to the girl in her ordinary clothes with no flower in her pot as his future bride. The other girls just couldn't understand why he chose the girl without a flower.

"I chose her," said the prince, "because the seeds I gave you all six months ago were infertile and could never germinate and bear flowers. The girl of my choice never pretended to be anything she wasn't, and she remained honest. A true queen."

(Inspired by a traditional story recounted by Paulo Coelho in his book *Stories for Parents, Children and Grandchildren*)

Talking in the Circle

After a story reading, have the children sit in a circle facing each other and have them discuss what the story meant and the message it carries. The story about the princess is inspired by a story by Paul Coelho and tackles the subject of honesty. Ask the children for examples of times they were honest, even when they were scared to be.

When discussing philosophy, let the children themselves speak as much as possible. As an adult, don't give them answers or make judgments about what they say. Not everything needs to be discussed. A single question may be enough to get a discussion going. If the discussion starts to wander off topic, ask another question to do with the story. Of course, the children may have questions of their own.

The message of the stories is that whatever people do will come back to them. If someone is honest, sincere, loving, and considerate, then that is what he or she will get from others in return. The saying "do unto others as you would have them do unto you" is a golden rule of yoga.

Experiences with Crystals

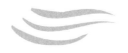

These stories introduce children to the world of crystals. Crystals are often used for their healing powers and as jewelry. For children, they seem to hold some wonderful magical power.

Crystals are mysterious because they have come out of the bowels of our planet. Long ago when the earth was still developing, crystals were dissolved in water. Later, they crystallized into beautiful shapes and colors. In the depths of the earth, crystals often look like lumps of uninteresting gray rock. Yet if you break the stone open in the sunlight, the wonderful forms and colors come to life.

The crystals are introduced with stories about Su. Su is a young girl who imagines that she has the most wonderful adventures on a magic bearskin. She flies all over the world on her bearskin and visits her invisible friends. The stories can be read together or separately.

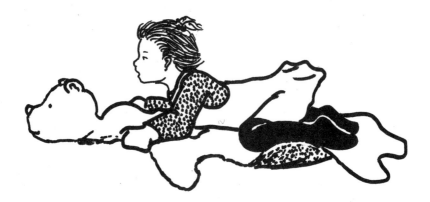

The Crystal Cave

Read the story to the children. Ask them to share their ideas about it afterward.

Su lies on her bearskin rug and whispers, "Dear bearskin rug, fly, fly, fly!" Today the bearskin rug flies Su to the crystal cave. In the middle of the cave is a huge piece of rock crystal. There is a wonderful blue light hanging there. In the walls, precious stones and crystals of every color of the rainbow twinkle and glisten. Su says, "I have never seen anything so beautiful."

A gleaming transparent Crystal man comes up to Su. He greets her: "I am the crystal man. I see you are admiring our wonderful crystal. The stone men live inside. The stone men make sure that crystals grow all over the world in caves and grottos and in the crevices in the rocks. We cut and polish them with love so that the light from the crystal can shine into the world. Our job is to give the rock crystal six sides and a point at the top. We're only happy when it looks like a crown or the roof of a castle! The most difficult thing is to burn in the rainbow colors. We use little flames to burn the seven colors into the crystal. The colors are red, orange, yellow, green, blue, indigo, and violet. If you hold the crystal up to the light, it will show you its colors."

The crystal man leads Su to another part of the cave to meet his three brothers. Their names are Smoky Quartz, Amethyst, and Citrine. The Citrine man skips up to Su and says, "I am the brother of the rock crystal. I have a yellow coat. Look—I shine like the Sun! The sunlight is caught inside my crystal. I help people get rid of their sad thoughts. If you carry citrine in your bag, your heart will jump for joy and your mood will be as light and bright as the Sun."

Then the purple Amethyst comes and bows deeply to Su. "Hello Su, I am so glad you came!" The Amethyst man speaks slowly with a deep voice like a king. He says, "I am a good stone for sleeping. If you put me under your pillow, you will sleep soundly and have wonderful dreams. I am also very good for headaches. If you roll me back and forth across your forehead, I will magically take your headache away."

Now it is the turn of the Smoky Quartz man. His crystal coat glistens gray-black. He greets Su and introduces himself. "I am also a member of the crystal family. I grow in the deep caves in the mountains. If you have a stomachache, it helps to put a piece of smoky quartz on your stomach."

Now that they had all introduced themselves, the Crystal man and his brothers stand in a circle with Su. Together, they dance the dance of the rocks.

80

The Mothers
of the Mountain Crystal

Read the story to the children. Ask them to share their ideas about it afterward.

The Crystal man and his brothers bring Su to meet their seven mothers: Agate, Onyx, Jasper, Carnelian, Tiger's Eye, Rose Quartz, and Opal. The stone mothers live at the end of the crystal cave. Su looks at the women in wonder: seven mothers, would you believe it?

The first one to introduce herself is mother Agate. "My name Agate comes from a river on the island of Sicily called Achatis. That was the first place people found me." Mother Agate's robe glistens in a whole array of colors from light brown to dark brown, gray-blue, reddish, mother of pearl, white, and black. Agate says to Su, "You know, Su, the dwarves carve the most beautiful patterns in my stone. If you hold me in your hand, I can make you feel safe. I protect all life and give courage and power."

Now mother Onyx in her deep black robe speaks, "Hello Su. I am a black stone. If you hold me in your hand, against your ear, or on your head, you can hear all the sounds of the world. Holding onyx in your hand will help you to better hear the stories people tell you. If you have an earache, I can help you. Put the stone on your ear, and the pain will vanish."

Now it is the turn of mother Jasper. She greets Su: "Hello, I am mother Jasper. The stone men sometimes call me the Mother of all Stones. I wear different robes. One of my favorites is the red-brown color of the earth, but I also love wearing the green one with red flecks. If you hold me in your hand often enough, I will improve your sense of smell. Your nose will be able to discern many more scents. You will be able to smell the flowers, the earth, the trees, and the animals—but also everything that smells bad."

Mother Carnelian says, "My color is a shining orange-red that creates a wonderful transparent glow. If you hold me in your hand, I will connect you with the beauty of the earth and with everything that grows. I will improve your concentration and enhance your enjoyment of the wonders of life. If you hold me, you will feel the warmth radiating from me into you. Your fingers will become more sensitive and perceptive."

And here comes mother Tiger's Eye. "My mantle is striped golden yellow and golden brown. If you move me back and forth, you can see my pattern of waves. It shines like satin and changes constantly. The waves move like everything in life moves. If you place me on your stomach, I will fill your whole body with warmth. I will help you get rid of colds quickly. With a tiger's eye on your stomach, you can have the most wonderful flights of fancy."

Next is Rose Quartz. She introduces herself: "Dear Su, I am mother Rose Quartz. I have a very big heart that is full of love. Wherever I let my pink light fall, gentleness, tenderness, and love will grow. Whoever comes near me, I will cover with my pink robe. I open people's hearts to beauty. If you hold me in your hand or carry me in your pocket, all anger and jealousy will disappear, and you will become tranquil."

Finally, mother Opal introduces herself: "My name Opal means 'stone' in the language of ancient India. The special thing about me is that I can take on all the colors of the rainbow. Did you know that in every opal there is a drop of water?" She promises Su, "If you ever wear an opal as jewelry, I will send you an angel of happiness. If he comes to you, you will know it for sure."

Su's visit to the crystal cave is coming to an end. She embraces all seven crystal mothers and crystal brothers and bids them farewell. She thinks to herself, "I'm glad I have only one mother and only have to say goodbye once." Su steps back onto her bearskin rug and whispers, "Dear bearskin rug, fly, fly, fly!" And she flies back to the other side of the world.

Drawing Crystals

Props: Paper; crayons, colored pencils, or markers

After listening to the stories, have the children make drawings. They might want to draw the crystal cave with the crystal man and his three brothers. Others might want to draw the seven mothers of the mountain crystals. Suggest that the children draw a rainbow, since rainbows show the colors that emerge from the crystals.

Feeling Crystals

Props: A variety of different crystals

Have the children sit in a circle around a bowl of crystals. Tell them to take turns picking up the crystals and holding them. They should feel the shape and the weight of the crystals.

After the children are finished feeling the crystals, help them to discuss what they discovered. Ask them if the crystals are warm or cold. What did the crystals have to tell them?

The Games Arranged by Specific Categories

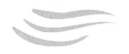

Games Requiring Props

37. Passing the Balloon
38. Teddy Breathing
46. Flower Meditation
48. Smelling
49. Hearing
50. Tasting
51. Feeling
52. Seeing
81. Drawing Crystals
82. Feeling Crystals

Games Not Requiring Props

1. Fingers
2. Wrists
3. Knees
4. Feet
5. Hips
6. Sun Salutation
7. Downward-Facing Dog
8. Cow's Head
9. Eagle
10. Turtle
11. Camel
12. Bird
13. Horse
14. From Caterpillar to Butterfly
15. Frog
16. Mouse
17. Owl

18. Shark
19. Penguin
20. Seal
21. Crab
22. Tree
23. Cobra
24. Elephant
25. Ape
26. Lion
27. Bear
28. Bending Sideways
29. Up and Down
30. Dangling
31. Wheelbarrow
32. Living Tunnel
33. Walking Numbers
34. Guessing Letters
35. Getting Knotted
36. Freezing and Melting
39. Balloon Breathing
40. The Breathing Ladder
41. Breathing with Sounds
42. Correct Posture
43. Sitting Still and Counting
44. Watching the Clock
45. Walking
47. Balloon Meditation
53. Bouncing
54. Stomping
55. Concave and Convex
56. Raising the Hips
57. Jumping
58. Pressing the Navel
59. Circles
60. Up and Down
61. Backward and Forward
62. From Right to Left
63. Shoulder to Shoulder
64. Elbow Butterflies
65. Rubbing the Crown
66. Warm, White Light

Games Requiring a Large Space

Games to Be Played in Pairs

Games to Be Played in Small Groups